ANATOMY

A STEP-BY-STEP GUIDE

ANATOMY

A STEP-BY-STEP GUIDE

Published by
Kandour Ltd
1-3 Colebrooke Place
London N1 8HZ
United Kingdom

This edition published in 2005 for
Bookmart Ltd
Registered Number 2372865
Trading As Bookmart Ltd
Blaby Road
Wigston
Leicester LE18 4SE

Author and Illustrations: Emmett Elvin
Managing Editor: Emmett Elvin
Cover Design: Alex Ingr
Page Layout: Emmett Elvin
Production: Karen Lomax

© Kandour Ltd

Printed and bound in India

ISBN: 1-904756-44-1

CONTENTS

INTRODUCTION

HOW TO USE THIS BOOK

For years, up until my late teens I would draw countless numbers of people, fuelled only by my imagination and what I thought I knew about the human body. As long as I was relatively uncritical of the shortcomings of my character's anatomy and those around me shared my reluctance to criticize, I could get away with it. If I hit a snag, I would simply find some quick fix reference, usually by referring to one of my favorite artists' work, and use this to get out of jail. Then one day I had a problem I couldn't fix. Not only that, but my favorite artists couldn't fix it either. I was in big trouble. As much as I hated to admit defeat, there was nothing else for it: I was simply going to

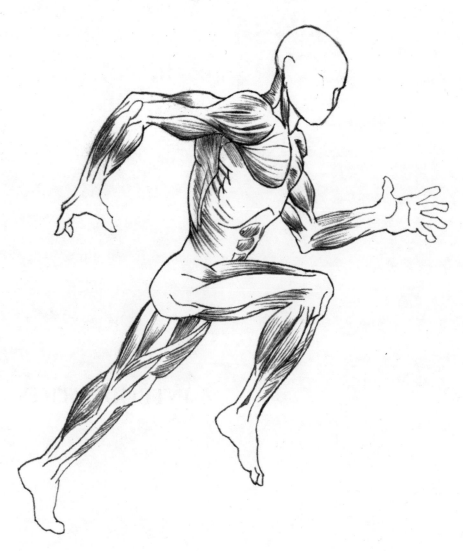

have to learn how the human body is really put together.

Talk about a humbling experience - I discovered to my horror how little I knew. About ten minutes later I also realized the power that this new knowledge would give me. To be able to draw any figure, male or female, young or old, skinny or voluminous

from any angle I pleased would really be a prize worth having.

Years later, and a mountain of books, illustrations and strips under my belt I'm still in awe of the mechanics of the human body. Amazingly, there is always something new to learn. Only recently I finally understood exactly how the tendons of the hand work in unison to fully articulate the fingers - the design of this feature of the body is particularly mind-blowing: perfection of design and purpose personified.

When planning this book I asked myself the same question I always do at a book's outset: "what kind of book would I have wanted when I was starting out?" To address this question I came up with the following criteria: that clarity and ease of understanding should at all times take precedence over beautiful or technically fantastic drawings. To this end I've tried to make sure that when you look at the illustrations in this book you know exactly what's going on and are able to resolve your own drawing problems.

A note on the latin names: it's not essential to learn off by heart all of the latin terms used to describe the anatomical parts herein. There are two good reasons for trying though: the first is simply as a memory aid - applying a name to

anything helps us remember. The second is that you may at some point find yourself discussing anatomy - at which point it's a good idea if both parties know the terms!

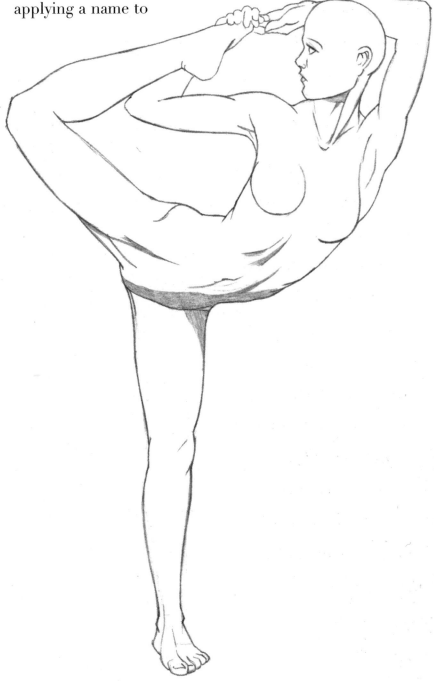

There are obviously going to be differences between a medical anatomy book and one that is intended for use by an artist. In this book I've deliberately left out organs, the arterial system, glands etc as these would be of little practical use for the artist. There are a few minor simplifications of muscle systems where , for reasons of clarity I've chosen not to show very minor muscles which have little or no chance of showing themselves on the surface of the body. Ultimately it *is* the surface of the body which the artist is concerned with and to this end I've included everything which can safely be said to influence the surface form.

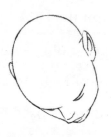

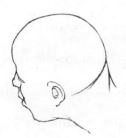

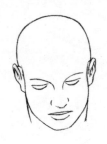

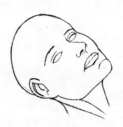

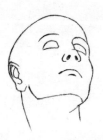

To really get the most out of this book you should use it in conjunction with some real life drawing. When we draw from life we're constantly being confronted with the unexpected, aspects of the human form that we would have little chance of successfully predicting without actually observing. It may not always feel as if we're learning from this process, but I honestly believe that every life drawing session we do contributes something to our understanding, even if we don't realize it at the time. Often this information will lurk in the back of our minds for years before it is drawn on, and we won't even necessarily realize it!

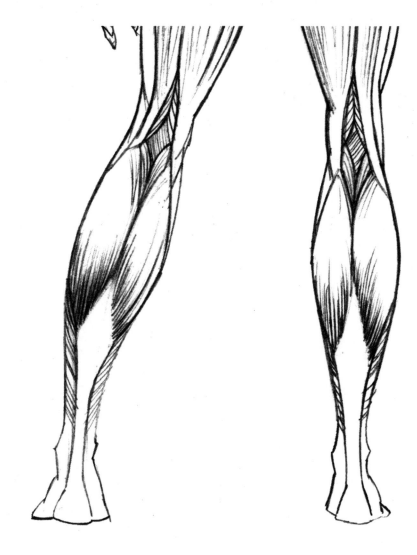

Another thing that life drawing can do for us is force us to look at the body from an angle we wouldn't necessarily think to draw it from. Ultimately, we're looking to build up a complete three-dimensional 'map' of the human form in our minds. Every unconventional angle we draw from will help us put this together. If you look at the drawings of the hands on page 89 you can see a good example of this. They are not drawn at the usual angle we think of when we think hands. As a result, they give us new and important information about their form.

This book has been constructed to enable the reader to either work their way through section by section or to dip into

to solve an immediate problem. Every chapter has the same structure: skeleton, muscle, surface, so by the time you reach the final chapter you should have a good idea of how the convergence of these three levels come together to produce the real life human forms found on those pages.

I've also included some exercises in planning your drawings. These are there to help you minimize the chances of losing control over a drawing.

Enough talk - let's get on with it!

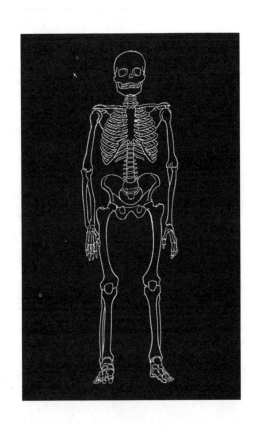

BODY

OVERVIEW OF THE HUMAN BODY
1: THE SKELETON

Thanks to ghost stories and horror films, all of us from an early age have at least a passing understanding of the framework of the human body. But how many of us know that an animated skeleton, even with supernatural intervention is an impossibility? Without ligaments and tendons holding the bones together the skeleton would be nothing but a pile of 179 bones on the floor! The joints of each bone are constructed according to their function. Ball-and-socket type joints are used where a high degree of freedom of movement is needed. More restricted hinge type joints are used where less freedom is required.

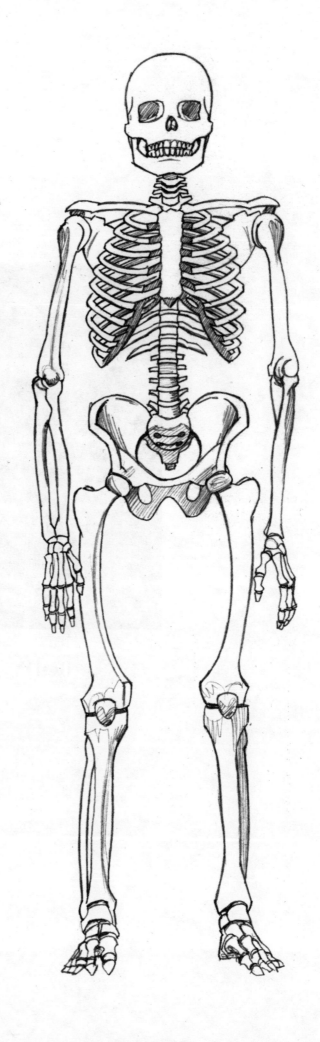

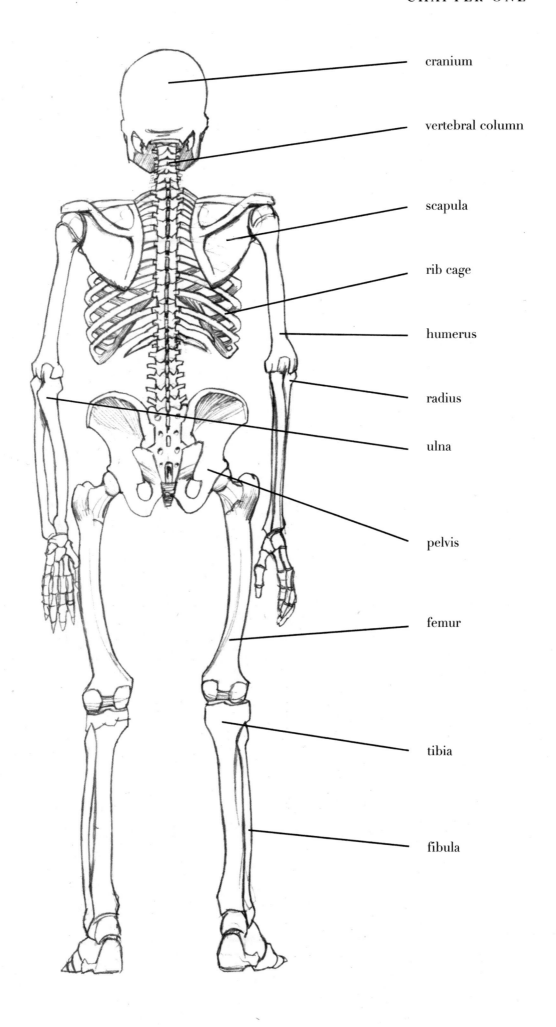

cranium

vertebral column

scapula

rib cage

humerus

radius

ulna

pelvis

femur

tibia

fibula

WHAT IS A BONE?

Every bone has numerous functions.

Its inflexibility allows it to effectively support the body parts directly above it. For instance, in the case of the ankle, this will involve a whole 'chain' of several bones going all the way to the cranium.

A bone also allows its surface to be used as an attachment point for ligaments and tendons, which in turn help articulate the body. Bones have a wide variety of notches, protrusions and what are called *tuberosities*; raised or bumpy areas of bone ideal for holding tendons or ligaments in place.

A bone additionally has to articulate with its neighbour. The degree to which it does this can vary from almost unlimited to almost nothing.

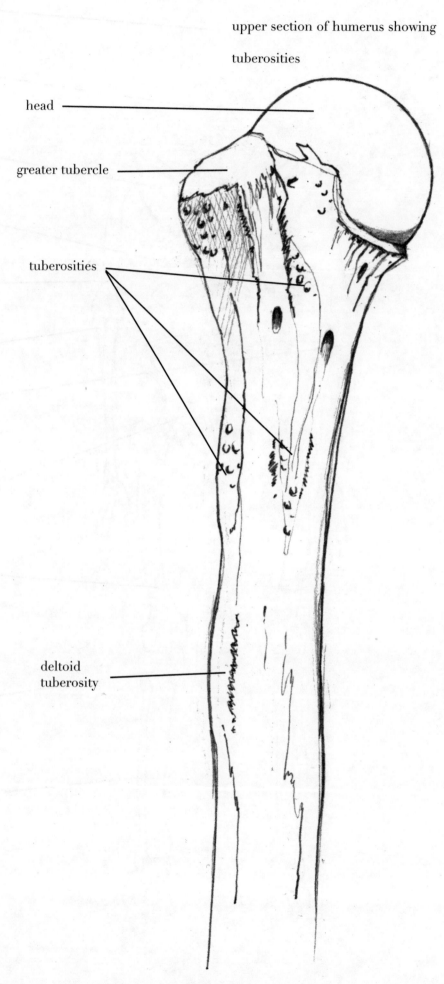

upper section of humerus showing tuberosities

head

greater tubercle

tuberosities

deltoid tuberosity

LIGAMENTS

Below is a simplified anterior view of the shoulder joint. The whole structure is encased in

Ligaments also play a large part in restricting us from actions such as hyper-extension and hyperflexion. This means

stretch or even tear one, as many people involved in the more physical sports will attest. Ligaments also play an

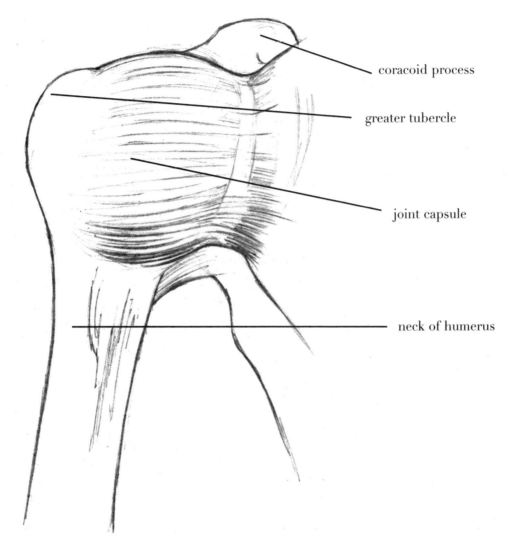

coracoid process

greater tubercle

joint capsule

neck of humerus

what is known as a joint capsule. This sheath of ligament serves not only to keep the joints together but is also lined with synovial membranes which keep the joint well lubricated.

stopping you from overreaching the limits of your body, which would otherwise result in torn muscle and other damage.

Tough as ligaments are, it's entirely possible to

important role in supporting various organs such as the liver and the uterus. They also play a large part both support and shaping of the breasts.

WIREFRAMES

For the sake of practicality, drawing an entire realistic skeleton as a framework every time we wanted to draw a figure would be both tedious and needlessly time consuming. For the sake of getting a figure up and running, we can instead turn to a greatly simplified version of the skeleton called a wireframe.

A wireframe allows us to map out the overall shapes and positions of the body parts quickly and efficiently. All the essential skeletal features are there, just represented in a more streamlined form. We can bring our knowledge of the real skeleton to bear when we're happy with the wireframe version, adding the 'real' features later on, where necessary.

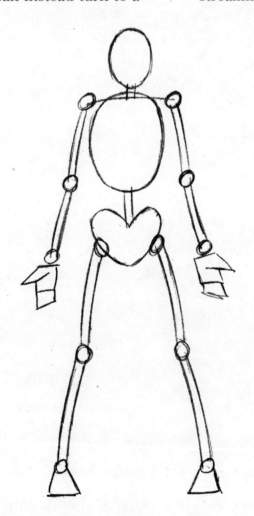

This wireframe has 'three dimensional' limbs. These can be useful especially for foreshortening.

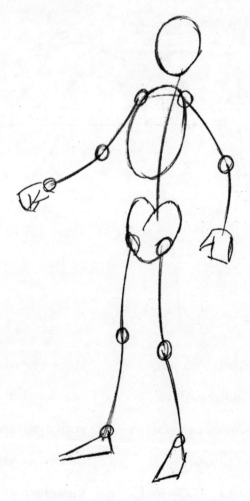

This wireframe is even more basic and is great for quick sketching.

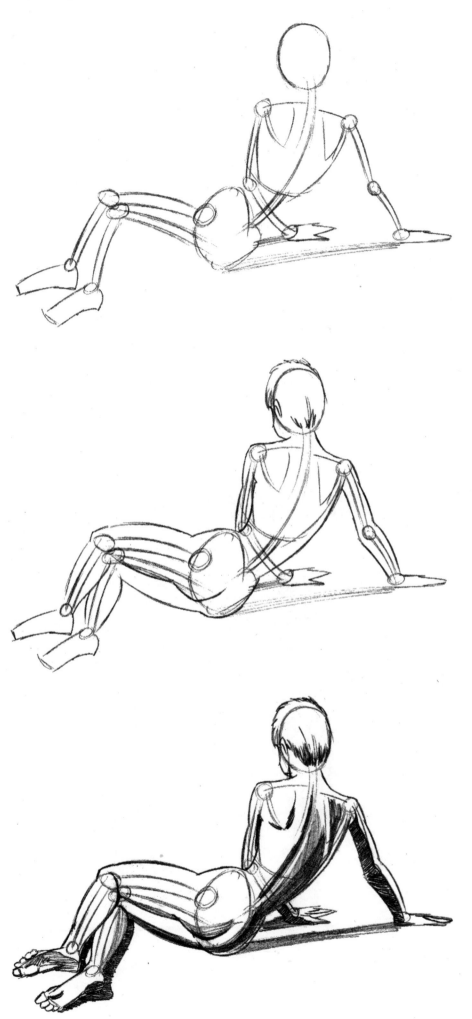

In this series of drawings we can see how this simplified skeleton or wirefrane can be used to help us plan a reasonably complex posture.

Notice at the point where the spine intersects with our model's left arm I've drawn both sets of lines. At this point we should 'draw through', which means to make sure all of the appropriate lines connect when it comes to finishing the job.

Next we flesh out the bones, adding body mass to the framework. No detail should be added yet.

The final stage is adding shadow and firming of detail etc. Normally we would clean up our guidelines prior to this, but I've left them in for the sake of instruction.

2: THE MUSCLE SYSTEM

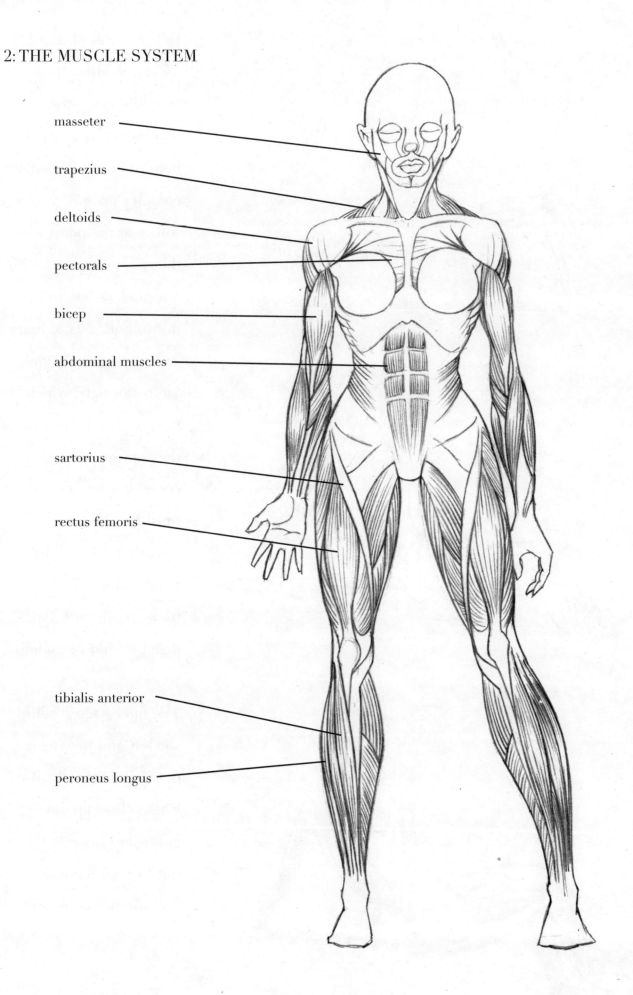

masseter

trapezius

deltoids

pectorals

bicep

abdominal muscles

sartorius

rectus femoris

tibialis anterior

peroneus longus

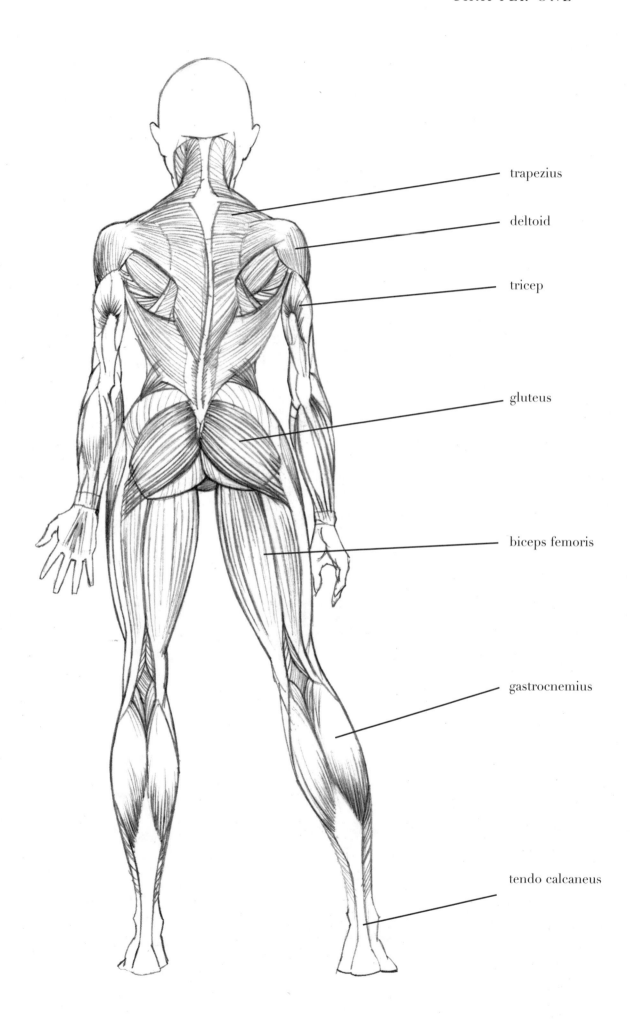

trapezius

deltoid

tricep

gluteus

biceps femoris

gastrocnemius

tendo calcaneus

WHAT IS A MUSCLE?

To the right is a typical muscle of the extensor or flexor kind. Extensor muscles are concerned with the straightening of a joint whereas the flexors are used for the bending of a joint. If you flex your bicep, you'll get a good idea of what a flexor muscle does. Conversely, if you straighten it out again to its full extent you'll find you're using your tricep muscles, a typical extensor type. This is illustrated even more graphically later on. All muscles have an origin, a function or action and an insert point. A typical origin point for a muscle might be the shoulder or other joint, although many muscles originate from the shaft of a bone, hidden deep below other

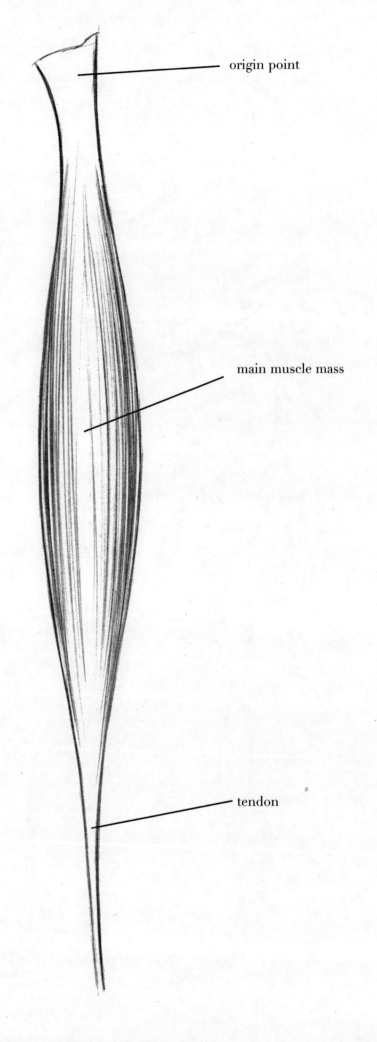

origin point

main muscle mass

tendon

layers of muscle. A muscle's action is dictated by its purpose. A key thing to remember is this: sections of the body are typically operated by the part above. The fingers of the hand are operated by the muscles of the forearm. Clench your fist for a moment and you'll quickly see the truth of this. To move your forearm upwards you'll need to use the services of your upper arm, specifically the bicep. And so on. Knowing this can help us make important artistic decisions about where to emphasize stress. Every drawing demands choices. The more informed we are, the better our choices are likely to be.

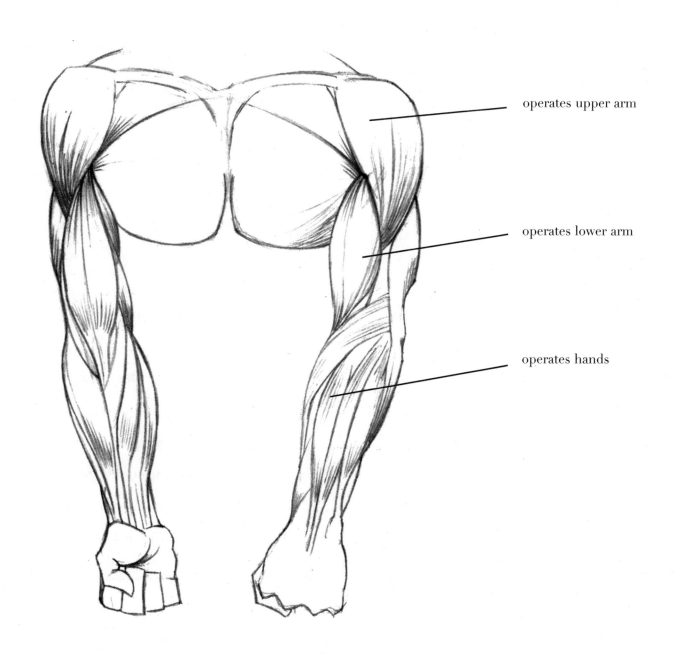

operates upper arm

operates lower arm

operates hands

USING WIREFRAMES TO DRAW DYNAMIC FIGURES

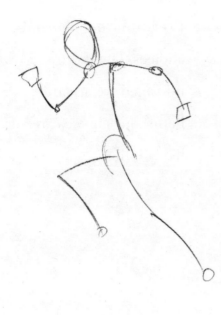

Let's use the principles of the wireframes first mentioned on page 18 to look at how we can use these effectively to capture the essence of a moving figure.

Figures in motion have a dynamic element to them not present in stationary models. Different muscle groups are brought into action and the human body can gain a form of expression that the standing or seated model simply never will.

Let's start with something comparatively simple - a running figure. The first strokes we make are both the fastest and the most important. To many readers, this may seem

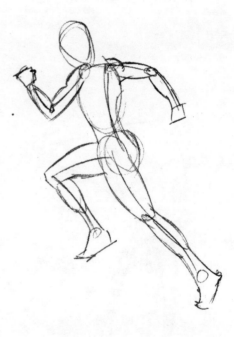

like a contradiction. Shouldn't we spend more time on the most important lines? No! We are trying to capture a moving figure. Slow, careful lines will likely result in a stiff or lifeless pose. To capture dynamics, we have to be dynamic in our approach.

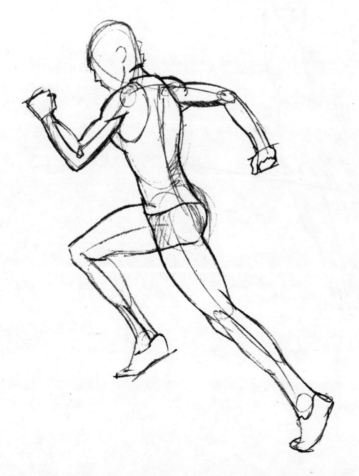

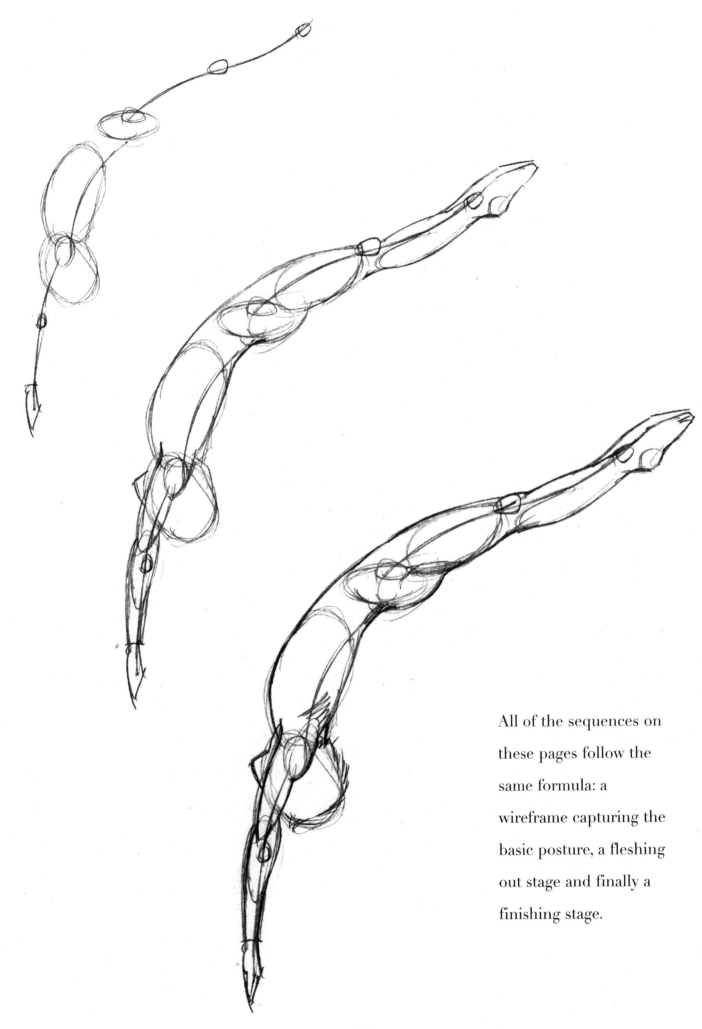

All of the sequences on these pages follow the same formula: a wireframe capturing the basic posture, a fleshing out stage and finally a finishing stage.

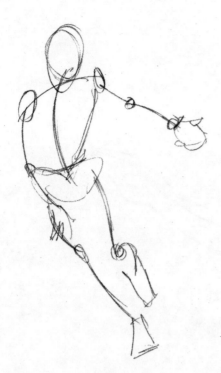

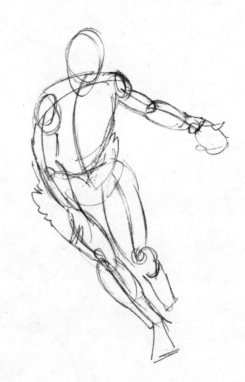

This figure of a basketball player is a good example of how to abuse the laws of weight in order to infer movement. We know that there is no way a person can possibly remain standing at this angle, so it can mean only one thing: that the figure is in the middle of shifting his weight as he makes his way across the court. However, we can only get away with this trick if our drawing is structurally convincing.

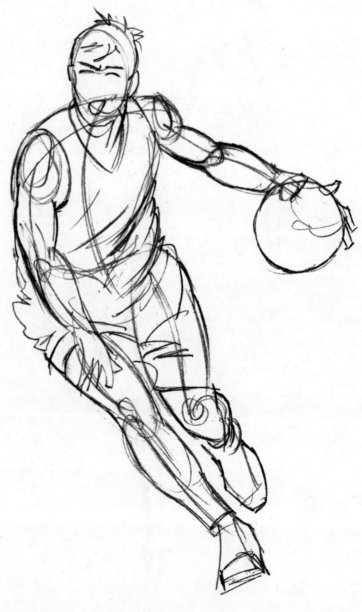

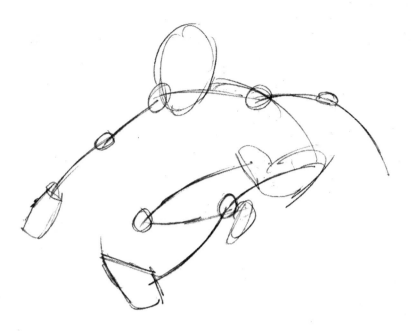

Let's give ourselves an even greater challenge by having a leaping figure, but drawn at a three quarter angle. The spine can be the hardest thing to wireframe due to it being foreshortened. Foreshortening has the effect of increasing the severity of any curve. If we work out where the base of the skull is and also the sacrum of the pelvis it should be a reasonably simple case of then connecting the two, making sure our spine has sufficient curvature.

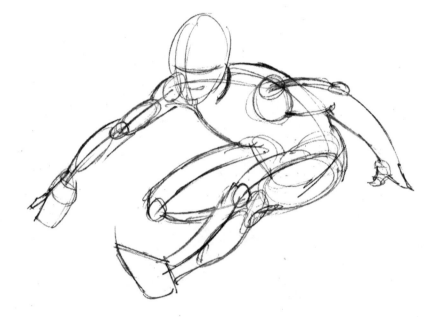

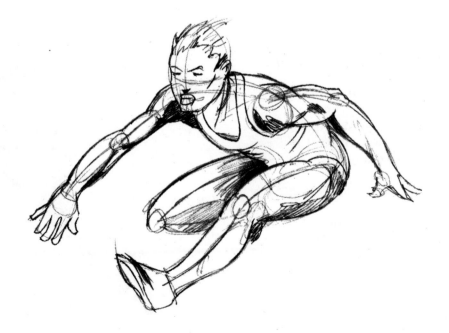

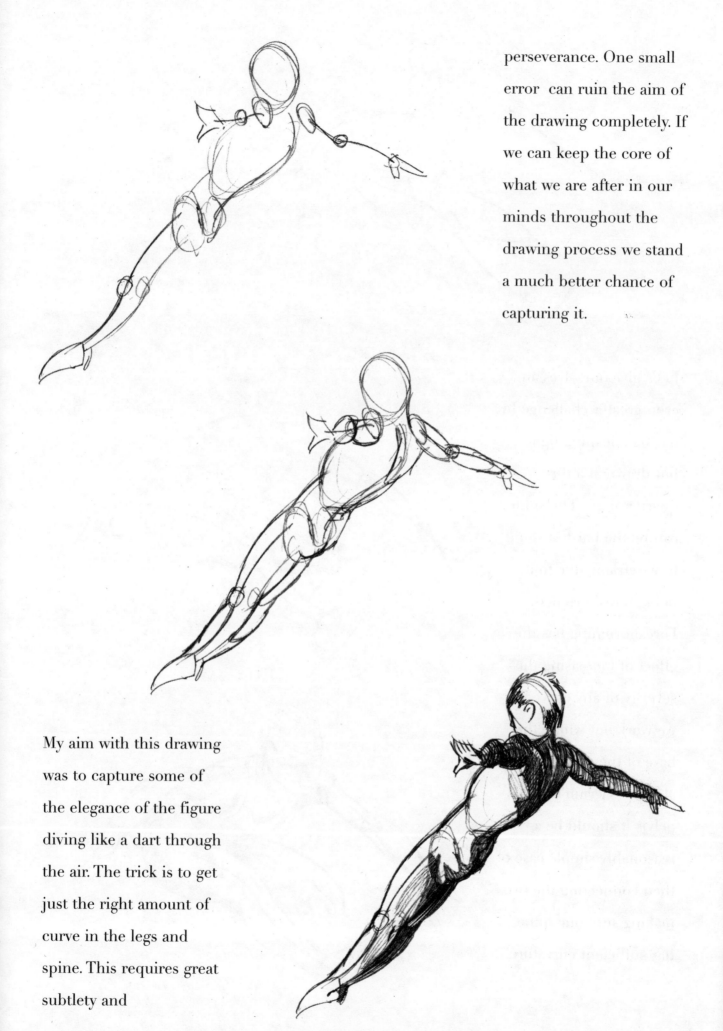

perseverance. One small error can ruin the aim of the drawing completely. If we can keep the core of what we are after in our minds throughout the drawing process we stand a much better chance of capturing it.

My aim with this drawing was to capture some of the elegance of the figure diving like a dart through the air. The trick is to get just the right amount of curve in the legs and spine. This requires great subtlety and

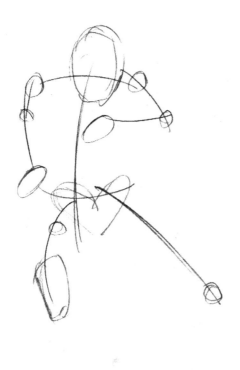

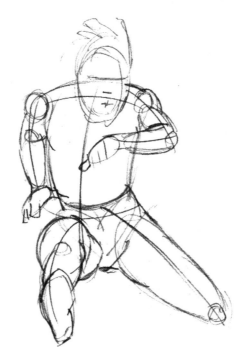

The second stage involves getting to grips with the foreshortening on the right leg. Foreshortened body parts tend in reality to be shaped quite unlike how we may expect them to be, so care and observation is key here. For the foreshortened left arm we need to make sure we put the upper arm in front of the shoulder.

Let's close with some extreme foreshortening. This hurdler's right leg is coming directly at the viewer while his left is pointing towards the ground.
The spine is straightforward in this wireframe. I've actually drawn it slightly to the left of where it should enter the pelvis, but rather than do the wireframe over, the rest of which I'm happy with, I'll compensate for it later.

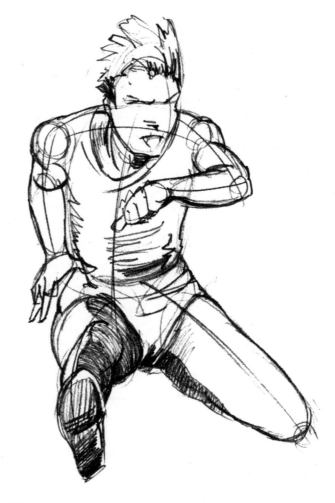

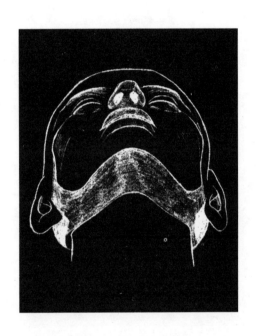

HEAD AND NECK

THE HEAD AND FACE

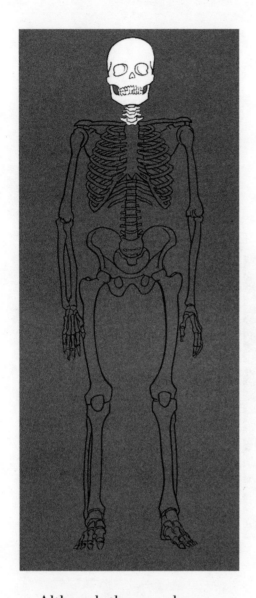

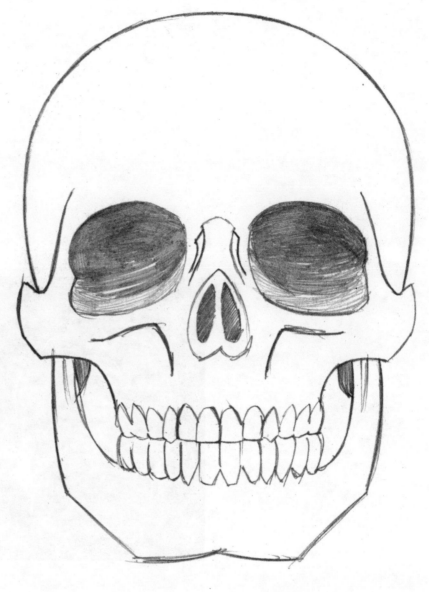

Although the muscles and skin play a part in giving a person their facial 'identity' it's the skull more than these that has the biggest influence on our facial features. Over time, peoples' skin changes, their muscles loosen, but they are still recognizable because of one thing - the unique shape and characteristics of their skull.

In a front view, the human skull is roughly at a ratio of 3 to 2, height to width. In a side view, the point where the mandible meets the cranium is a reliable halfway point.

Many people misjudge the depth of the cranium when they first begin drawing heads. Although there are 21 bones in the cranium, these are fused, making it practical to consider the skull as having only two bones: the cranium and the mandible.

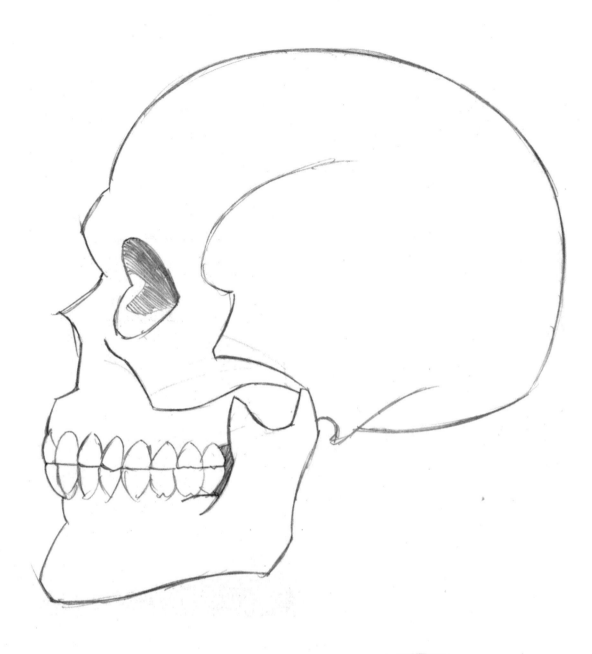

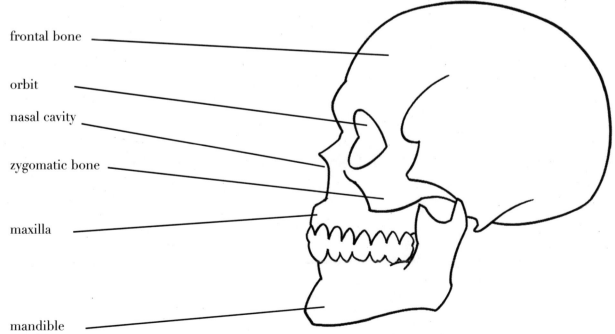

frontal bone

orbit

nasal cavity

zygomatic bone

maxilla

mandible

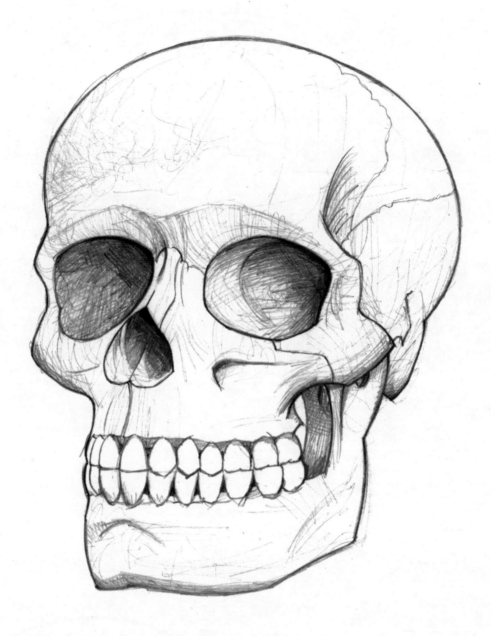

In the three-quarter view above we can more easily see the heavy protrusion of the *zygomatic* or cheek bones. This is a pivotal area to understand as many of the major muscles of the face arise from this area which as a whole is called the *zygomatic process*. The largest muscle of the face, the masseter originates here and inserts at the mandible at the back of the jawline.

The roof, or vault of the skull is composed of four fused bones joined by sutures.

The orbits, or eye sockets are bone-walled cavities at the rear of which are the orbital fissures and optic canal. As the name suggests, these openings allow the eye and brain to communicate.

MUSCLES OF THE FACE

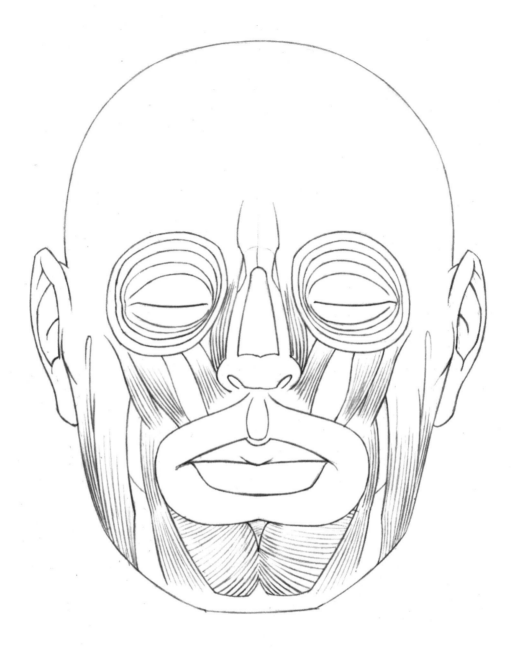

The muscles of the face are employed in a number of different functions. Chewing, blinking and a wide range of emotional responses are just a few examples. This is reflected in the great variety of muscles shown above.

As mentioned on the previous page the largest of these is the masseter, responsible for the function of chewing and biting. Clench your teeth and you will plainly feel these muscles at the back of your jawline.

The eye is surrounded by a ring of muscle called the *orbital oculi*. Forming the eyelids are the *palebral oculi*. The cheek muscles are comprised of *zygomaticus major* and *zygomaticus minor*, as well as the *levator labii superioris* muscles annotated overleaf.

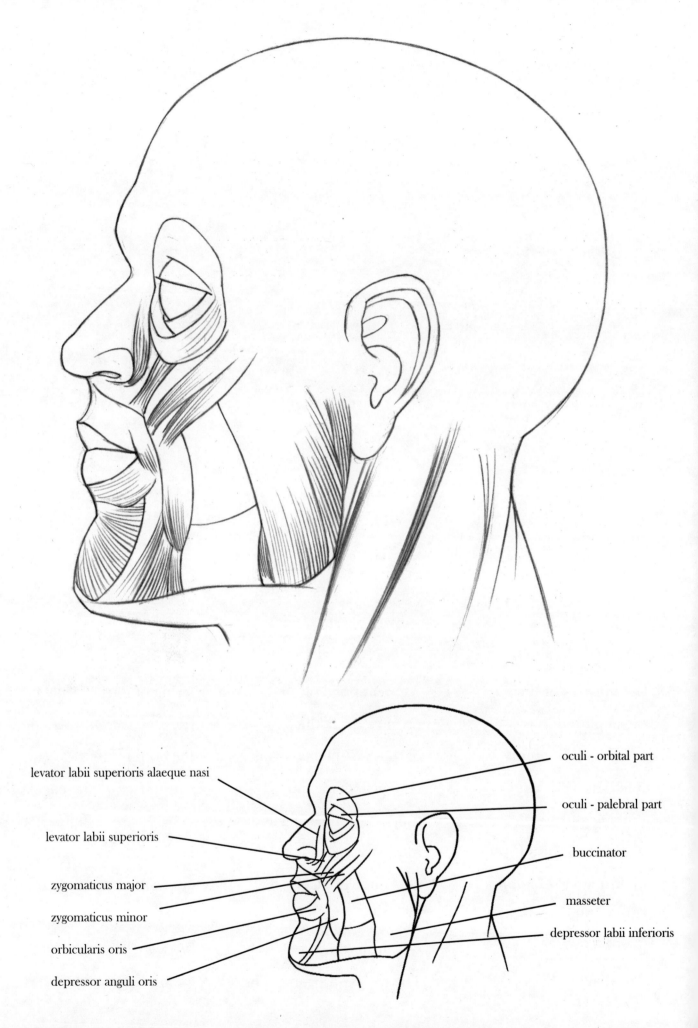

levator labii superioris alaeque nasi

oculi - orbital part

oculi - palebral part

levator labii superioris

buccinator

zygomaticus major

masseter

zygomaticus minor

orbicularis oris

depressor labii inferioris

depressor anguli oris

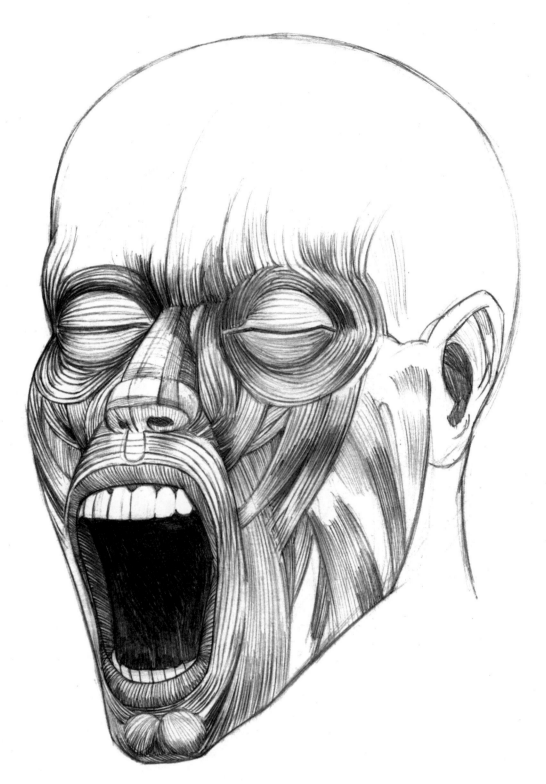

Above is an illustration showing the muscles being used to open the mouth to its full extent.

The *depressor labii inferioris* have become hardened and compressed in this action.

This pair of muscles are primarily employed in moving the bottom lip, so if the bottom teeth are showing in a subject it's almost a certainty that these muscles will be being used.

Although the masseter is being used to lower the jaw, it is not being used as a clamp, as in biting, thus the muscle mass at the jawline does not protrude.

The drawing on the left is a composite of the skull and the muscles of the face. In it we can better see the relationship between bone and muscle. We can for instance clearly see the zygomatic muscles emanating from the cheekbones and moving down the face toward their insertion point beneath the orbicularis oris.

There are two areas that are in fact neither muscle or bone but are made of cartilage, a tough, flexible material somewhat plastic in quality. At the point where the nasal cavity ends there is a section of cartilage joined to it called the septum. This keeps the nasal passages supported whilst allowing a good degree of flexibility.

The other cartilaginous

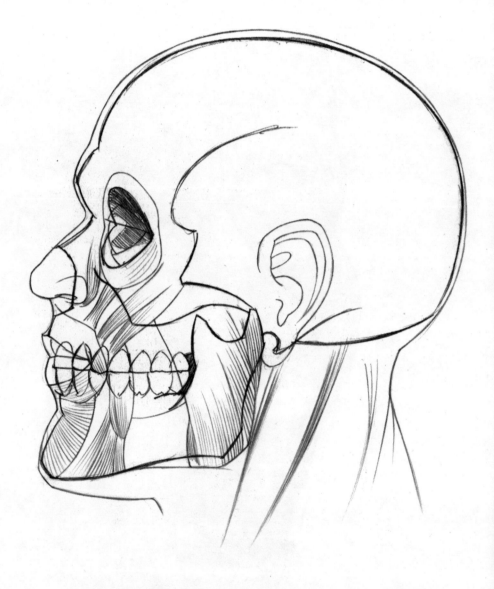

area is the ear. Like the septum of the nose, the ear has to be both flexible and durable, but has no real need to be mobile. The smaller features of the head that protrude are vulnerable to injury. Flexibility makes them able to deal with the knocks and strains that life is likely to bring to bear.

Cartilage provides the ideal material for this.

YOUNG FACE

With a young person's face the skin is tight and shows little or no lines beyond those typically found on a baby's. There is a roundness and predictability to the features. The ears are quite small at this stage but continue to grow throughout life. This can be clearly seen by comparing the two images.

OLDER FACE

As the body ages, its ability to repair or replace damaged cells diminishes, causing a loss of tightness in the skin. This is particularly noticeable in the skin of the neck and at the sides of the mouth. Also, repeated use of the same muscles during facial expressions causes frown lines, laughter lines etc to be permanently etched on the features of an older person's face.

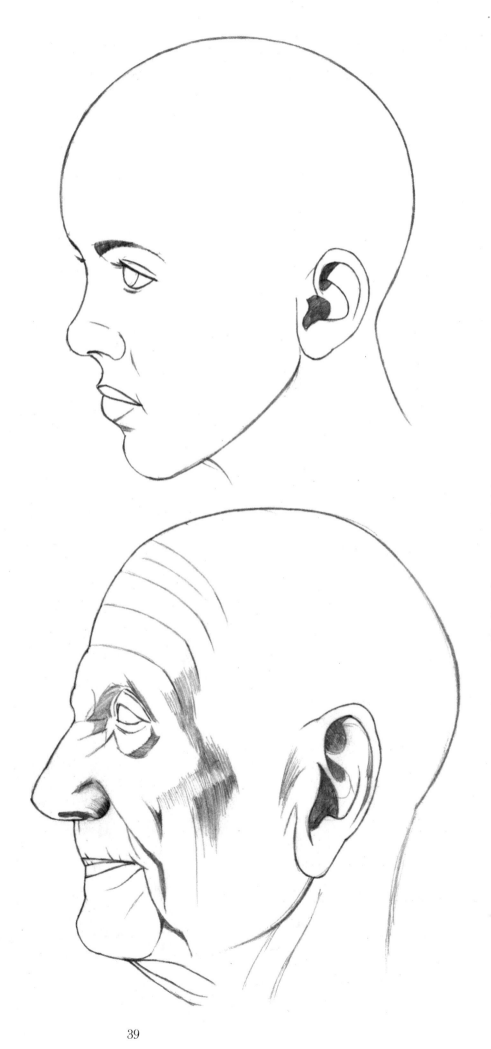

39

THE NECK

Below the jawline are a number of small muscles working in conjunction with a peculiar, very small bone called the *hyoid*. It is suspended from the temporal bones of the skull via ligaments and serves as an insertion point for several muscles of the throat.

The most prominent of the neck muscles when viewed from the front in real life are the mastoids, or *sternocleidomastoids* to give them their full latin name. These originate at the base of the cranium behind the ear where they are quite flat and wide. As they move towards the clavicle, their insertion point, they become more tubular before narrowing to tendons.

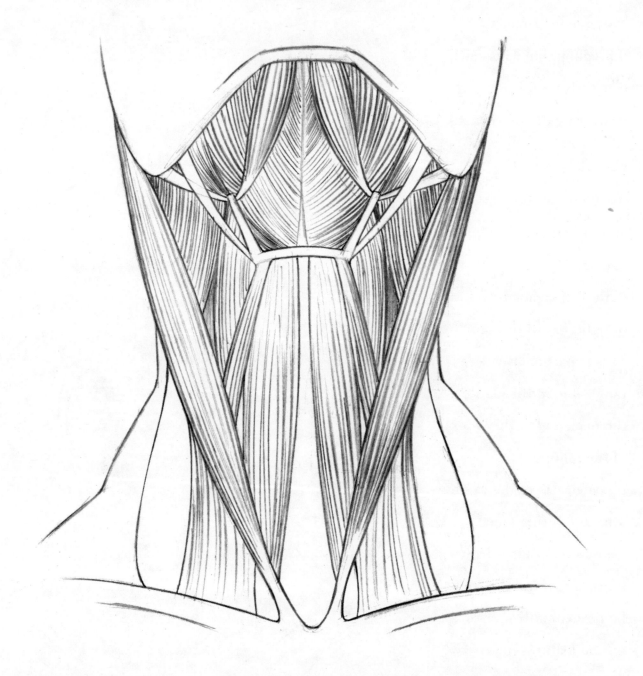

The principle function of the mastoid muscles is the turning of the head. It will also support the head if the whole body is tilted back.

If the head turns right the left mastoid will project outwards and vice-versa. The more extreme the head turn, the more pronounced the mastoid will become. This is a highly useful muscle for the artist as it is the one which most forcefully interacts with the torso.

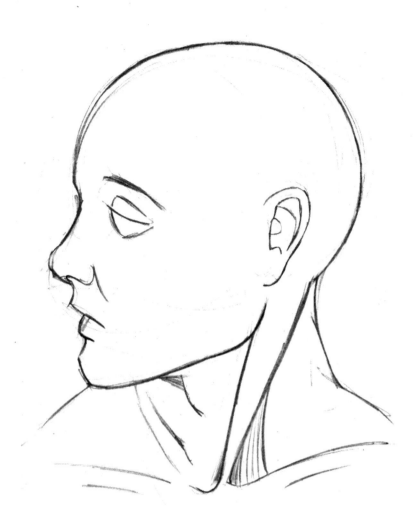

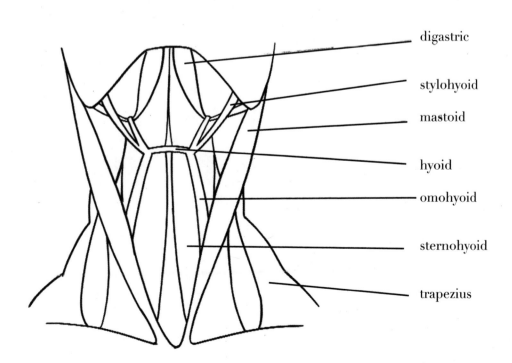

digastric

stylohyoid

mastoid

hyoid

omohyoid

sternohyoid

trapezius

41

REAL LIFE HEADS

The following pages show
how some simple
planning can ensure that
we always get our facial
features in the right
place, no matter how
oblique the angle we are
trying to draw.

We want ultimately to
have the ability to draw
the head in any position
and at any angle, but to
do this we need to have a
very strong mental
picture of the exact way
that the features move
through space when the
position or angle of the
head changes.

To achieve this, we don't
have to be able to
envision the precise
details of each feature,
only along which lines
those features will appear.
These three drawings to
the right show this
principle in a simple
form, using a three-
quarter angle.

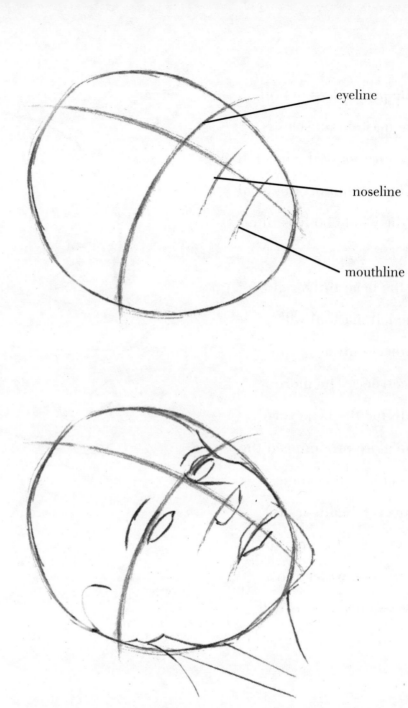

eyeline

noseline

mouthline

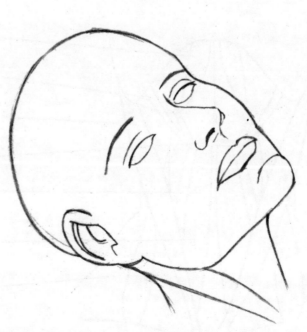

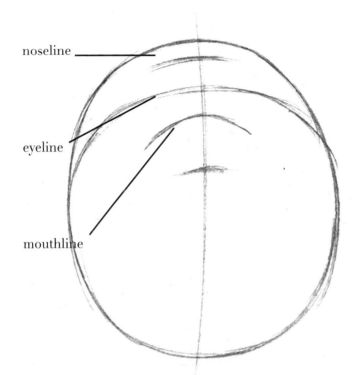

noseline

eyeline

mouthline

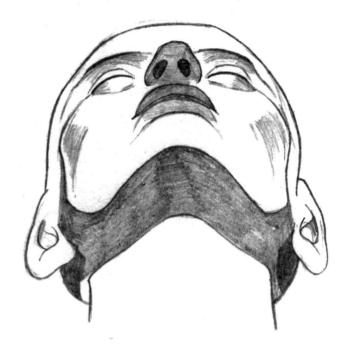

LOOKING UP:

The construction lines on all of these faces represent the eyes, nose and mouth. The order these appear, as well as the distance between them changes depending on the angle of tilt of the head. On the drawing above, the noseline is higher than the eyeline - the opposite of the previous page

LOOKING DOWN:

When looking down on a face, the eye, nose and mouth lines move down. The gap between the eyes and nose widens slightly and shortens between nose and mouth.

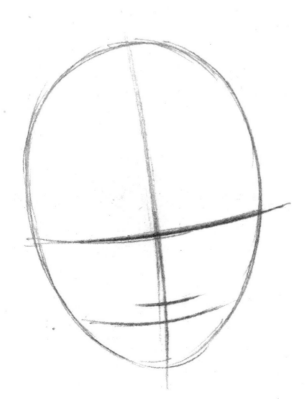

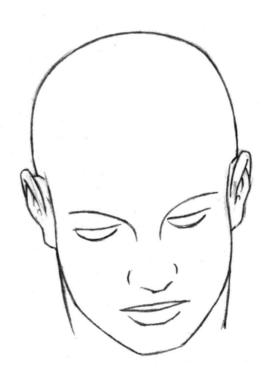

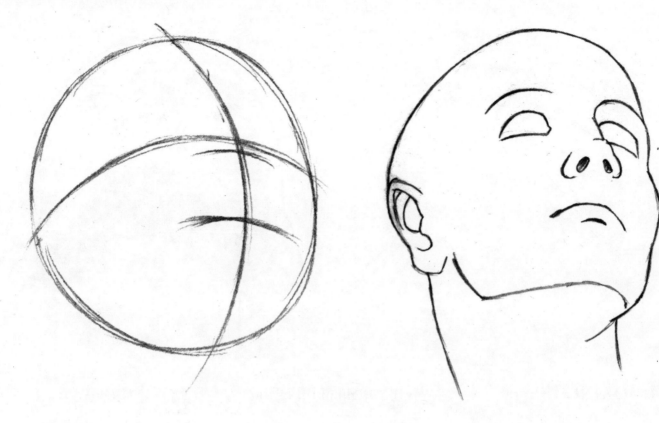

The above shows a head from a three-quarter angle, tilted back slightly and viewed from below.

Below is another view looking up, but with the mouth open. When fully open and viewed straight ahead, the mouth forms an 'o' shape with a greatly reduced distinction between upper and lower lips.

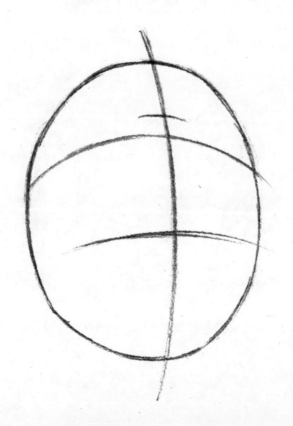

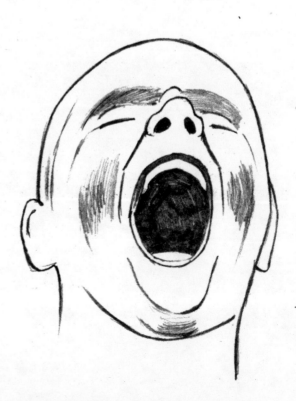

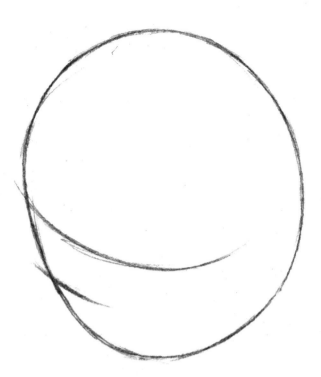

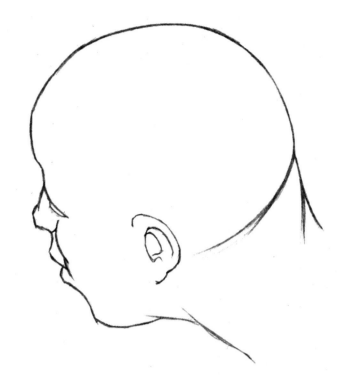

Needless to say, the most extreme oblique angles do not easily lend themselves to this formula. In these cases we simply have to map out what we can and improvise.

The extreme downshot is more straightforward: just remember the compression of the features is far more pronounced than in the drawing on page 43.

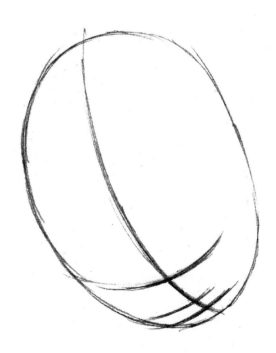

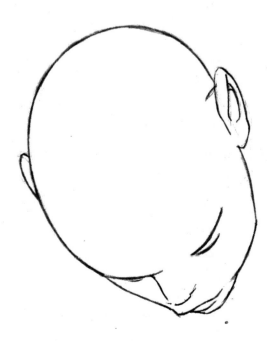

PORTRAYING EMOTION

Now that we've examined the muscles of the face and looked at ways to get our basic heads right, the next level is to consider the face as a means of expression.

The key to being in control of this is learning which nuances of expression are signifiers for the feelings being expressed. Just about every square milimeter of the human face expresses something, as we are about to see.

Because children's, and especially baby's faces are still quite structurally different to ours, they have an instinctive ability to convey expressions that an adult cannot compete with. Adults can look at something with awe, but a small child will

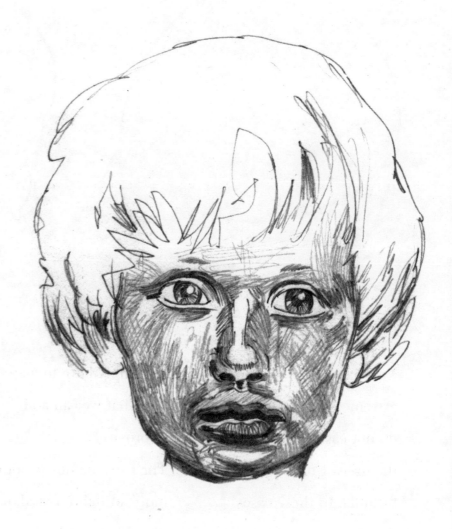

look at something in wonder.

Some of these signifiers, or facial nuances are common to expressions which are in direct opposition to each other. For instance, the folds around the mouth seen on the angry man opposite are also on the face of the blissfully happy girl on page 49.

Her eyes are also barely open and she has a 'knot' at the bridge of her nose, Just as Mr angry does. So why is one person looking like they are exploding with rage while the other is laughing their head off? The answer is that it is combinations of localized expression and not one lone factor that conveys the total emotional effect.

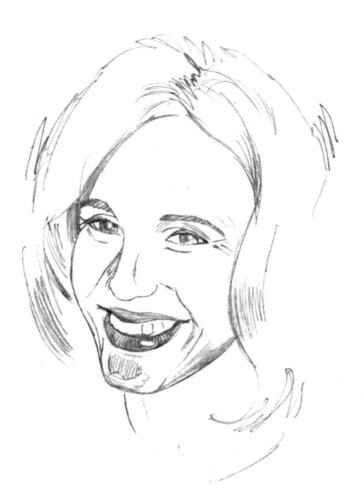

other minor signs of contraction of her oculi muscles. This is a description of a trademark happy face and as such comprises a 'shopping list' of the elements we would be looking for in order to capture that simple emotion.

The girl in the image above is wearing a typically cheery face. The edges of her mouth are turned up, her cheeks are lifted and her eyebrows are relaxed. The muscles of her depressor labii inferioris are projecting her chin outwards causing subtle lines to appear around the chin's margins. There is just a hint of 'crow's feet' around her eyes and

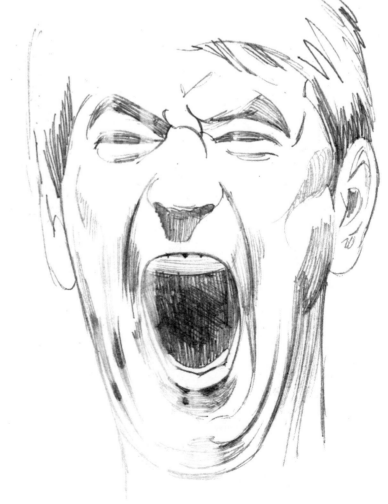

A worried or insecure face poses a very different challenge. Rather than the big, blatant expressions of the happy face, a mildly fearful person is more likely to have an expression which is the culmination of many subtle facial nuances. The eyebrows are slightly arched and

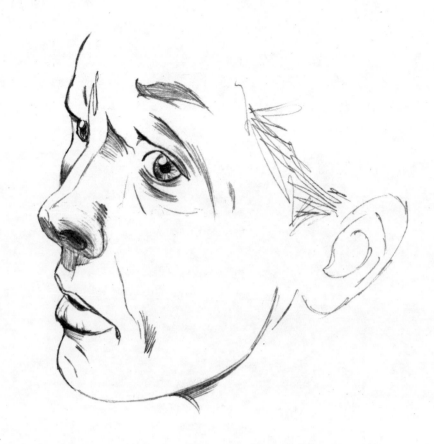

the mouth is slightly open - a surefire signifier of expected trouble on this type of face. The eyes will not mirror each other as a relaxed person's normally would but will appear to be behaving somewhat independently of each other. This helps to give them a 'haunted' look.

The extremely upset face of the man on our left shares the use of the *depressor labii inferioris*

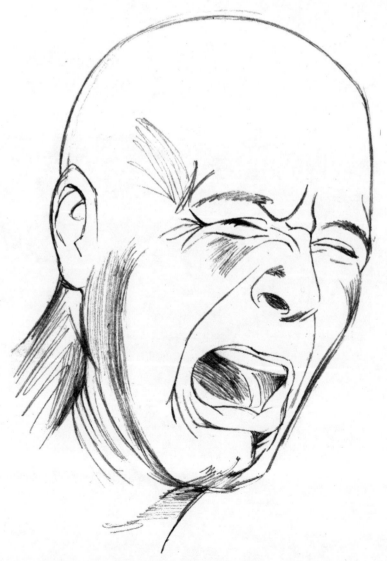

with the happy girl. But in this case, however the chin is being pulled in rather than being jutted out. This is a classic feature of the 'crybaby' face.

In deep grief, the nasal passages tend to flare and there is an extreme bunching of the thinner flesh around the eyes and the bridge of the nose.

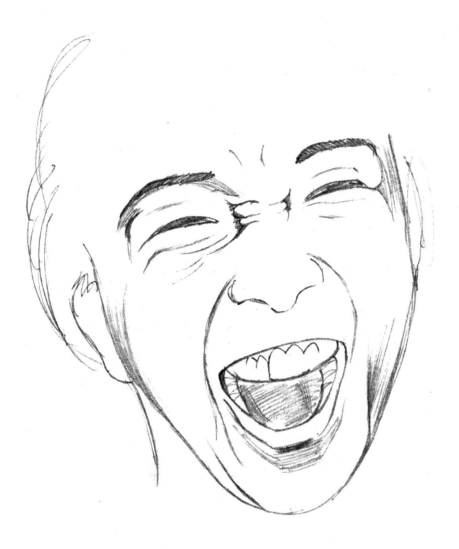

This tight bunching is also shared with our laughing girl here, as are the nearly closed eyes. However, she and Mr Misery share very little else. The corners of her mouth do not appear to be downturned and yet, she is obviously deliriously happy. Is some other feature contributing to her deep happiness?

The ultimate point of this type of analysis is not to then impose our own expressive wishes on a model. Rather it is about being able to make an informed choice about how best to bring the character out faithfully.

The human face is an ever-changing pool of emotional possibilities, with no hard divisions between one expression and the next. Humanity has found ways to express every emotion through the facial features. Understanding exactly how these are conveyed is a key part of our development as an artist.

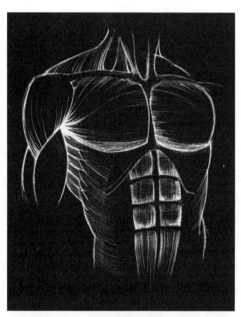

TORSO

THE SPINE

The spinal column and
the pelvis represent the
two most important
aspects of posture.
In the diagram below we
have a standing figure.
The figure looks balanced
and comfortable because
the posture is correct.

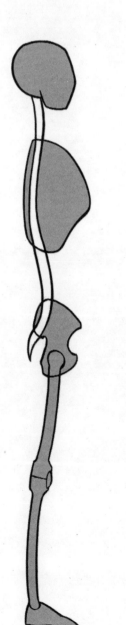

cervical curve

thoracic curve

lumbar curve

sacral curve

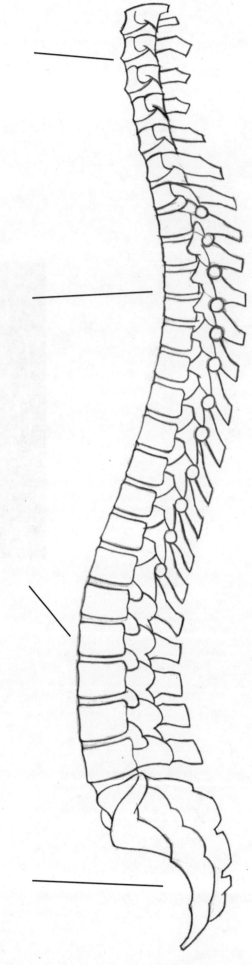

This is in no small part due to the correct curvature and positioning of the spine.

The spinal column has four areas of curvature as shown on the previous page. These four areas correspond to the neck, the rib cage, the lower back and the pelvis. The seven topmost vertebrae, beginning with the large *atlas* vertebra make up the neck. The following twelve form the thoracic section as these vertebrae are those having ribs joined to them. The most massive of the vertebrae are the five *lumbars* which in turn join the *sacrum*. This is essentially a fusion of smaller vertebrae forming one unit. It terminates at the *coccyx* and may or may not be fused with it.

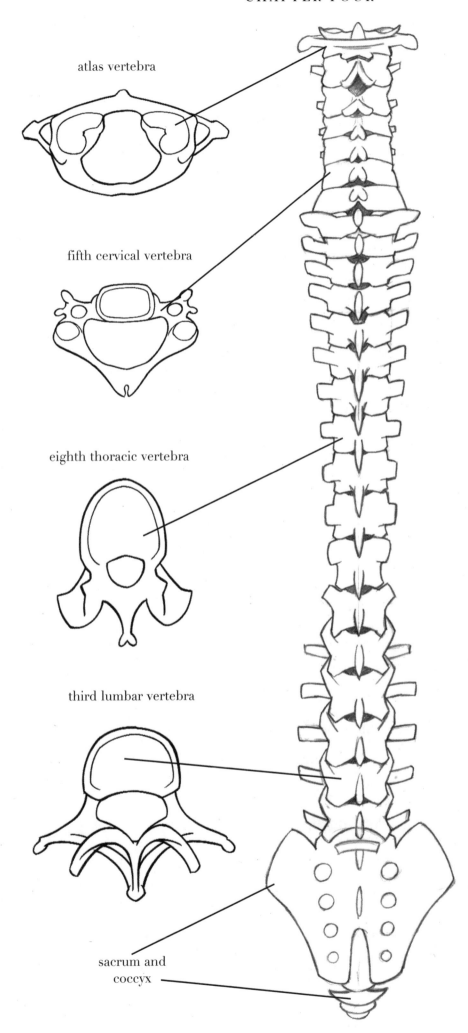

atlas vertebra

fifth cervical vertebra

eighth thoracic vertebra

third lumbar vertebra

sacrum and coccyx

SPINAL MUSCLES

Running the entire length of the spine are the *erector spinae* group of muscles. These support the spine from the coccyx to the base of the cranium. As most of this muscle group lies at a very deep area, much of it is only hinted at, with the expansive trapezius muscle overshadow it at the upper back region. It is, however, far less covered and thus more visible at the lower back where its characteristic shape can be made out quite easily. Typically, these muscles when used take the shape of a pair of cables straddling the spine and are particularly noticeable at the lumbar area when the back is arched or weight is shifted from leg to leg.

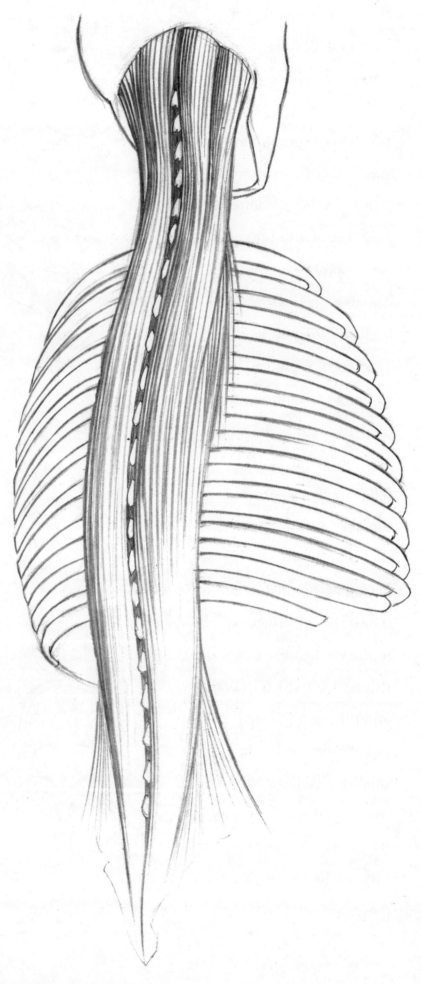

THE RIBS

Enclosing and protecting the heart and lungs are twelve ribs, divided at the front by the *sternum* and at the back by the spine. The sternum is a flat bone in two sections at the sides of which are notches which accommodate the ends of the first seven, or true ribs. These sections of rib are elastic and are called costal cartilages. They are what allow our rib cage to expand and contract as we breathe. Ribs eight to ten share their connection to the sternum and are referred to as *false ribs*. The bottom two are called *floating ribs* for the obvious reason that they are connected to the spine but not elsewhere.

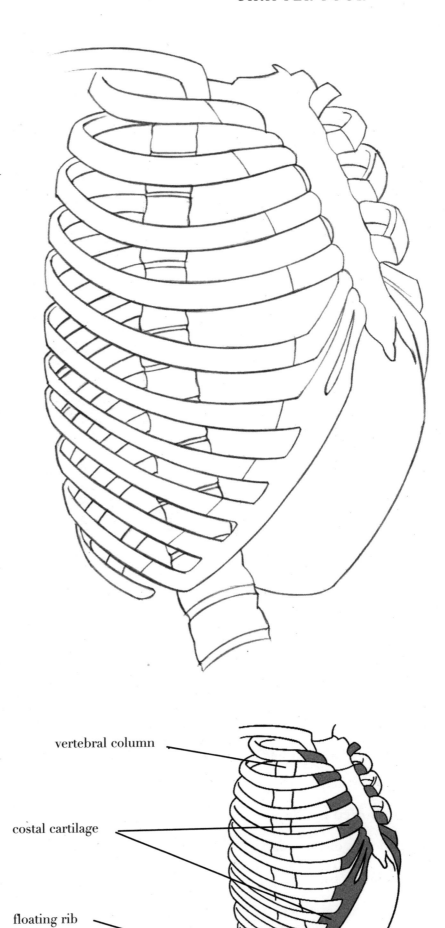

vertebral column

costal cartilage

floating rib

THE PELVIS

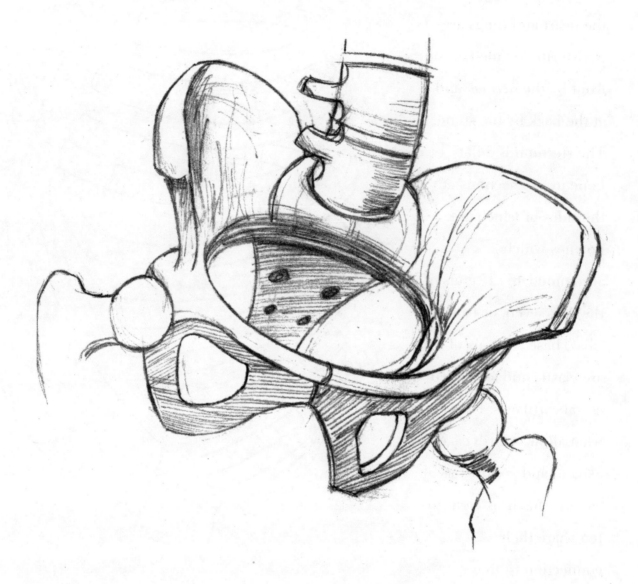

The hub of the body, the pelvis is a basin-shaped area supporting the torso and supported by the femur bones of the thigh. It has a wide, roughly circular opening at its base and a distinctive rising enclosure at its back and sides called the

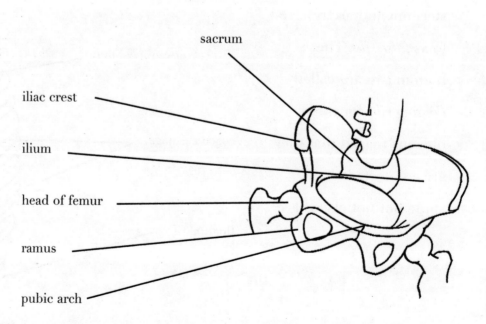

sacrum

iliac crest

ilium

head of femur

ramus

pubic arch

56

ilium, the ridge of which is the *iliac crest*. Put your hands on your hips and you will be resting them on this crest. At the rear of the pelvis is the sacrum, which has been mentioned before due to it's association with the spine. It is at this point that the spine joins the pelvis, as can be clearly seen on the facing page. Beneath the ridge and rim of the ilium is the *ischium*. Here we can see the distinctive mask-like shape of the ramus part of the ischium, clearly visible overleaf. The rami provide excellent origin points for several thigh muscles. The pubis is the third main section of the pelvis and forms the frontal or anterior rim . At the point where all three sections meet is the *acetabulum*, a large socket which houses the head of the femur and is clearly visible at the bottom left of the image below.

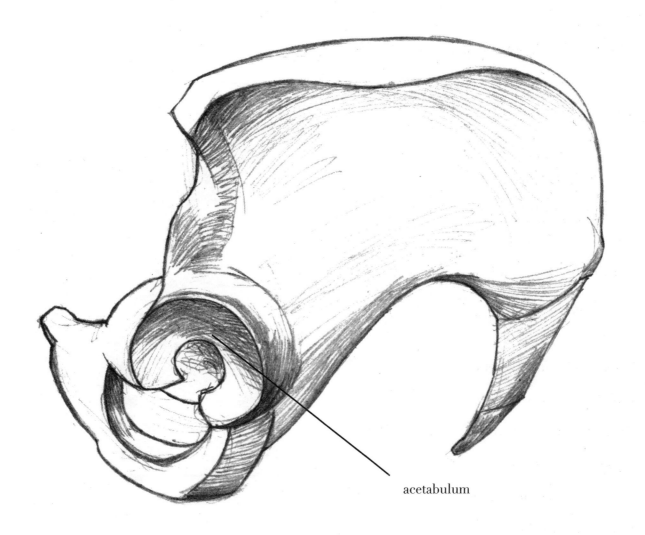

acetabulum

SERRATUS MUSCLES

This group of small muscles are often hidden from view by the arm. They have their origin at the base of the lateral side of the clavicle and attach themselves to the ribs as shown below. They are at their most prominent when being used to help raise the arm, but even then much of these muscles are obscured by the *latissimus dorsi*. This is a large, long and fairly shapeless muscle covering the area between the trapezius of the back and the serratus, and running down behind the back and attaching to the iliac crest of the pelvis.

These are a useful set of muscles to look for when drawing a torso as the majority of this area below the pectorals and to the side of the abdominals is largely lacking in identifying features. There is a large and extremely flat muscle area called the *obliquus externus* which interdigitates with the serratus, sweeping down towards the pubic area where it is lost under a deep aponeurosis covering the belly.

The drawing opposite shows this area and the aforementioned interdigitations. It is an area of no small complexity and mastery of it requires much study.

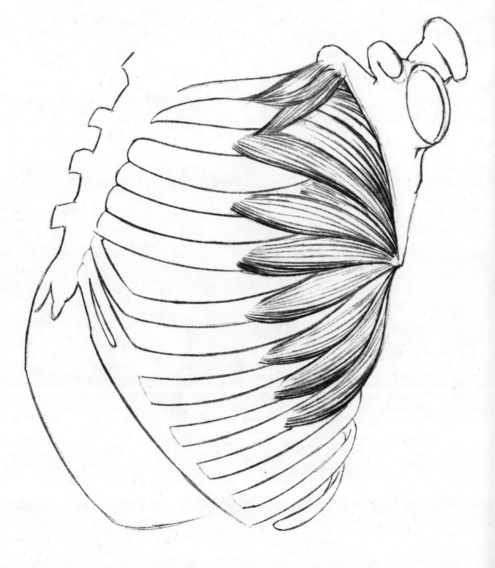

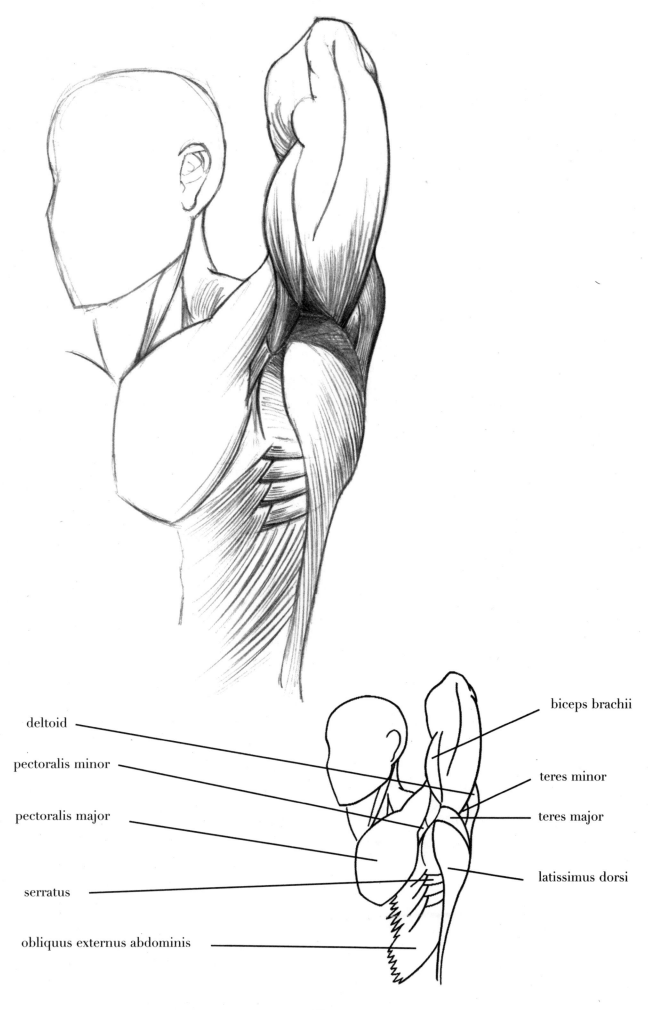

deltoid

pectoralis minor

pectoralis major

serratus

obliquus externus abdominis

biceps brachii

teres minor

teres major

latissimus dorsi

THE BACK

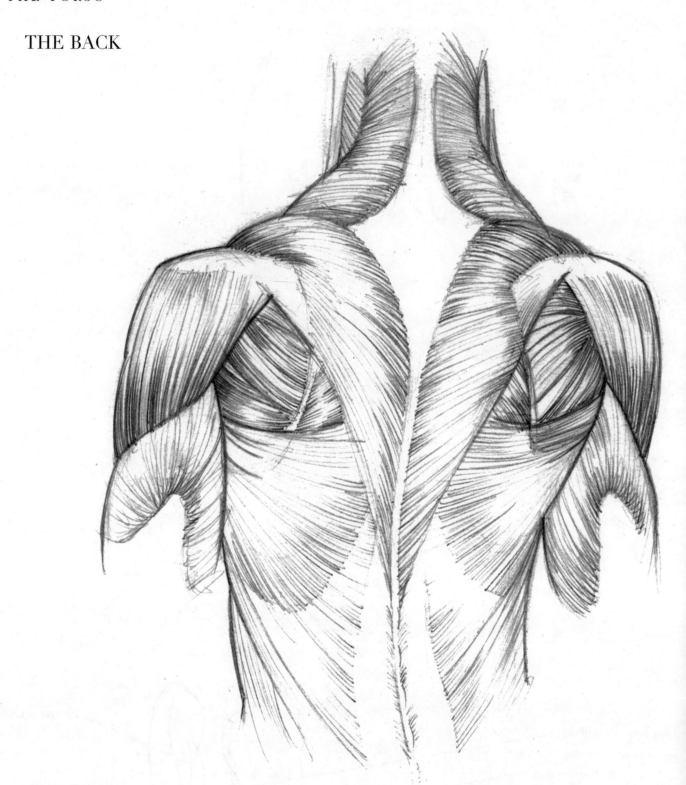

For the very reason that the back lacks the more blatant features of the front of the trunk it can prove difficult at first to gain a foothold in our understanding.

The most obvious muscles present here are the large, central ones, which form a diamond or trapezium shape at their centre, giving the *trapezius* muscles their name.

Between these and the deltoids are a group of muscles overlaying the scapula, the largest of which is the *infraspinatus*, a large but mostly deep layer of muscle. A section of *rhomboideus*, the majority of which lies below the trapezius can be seen here and the two *teres* muscles, *major and minor* appear here between the infraspinatus and latissimus dorsi.

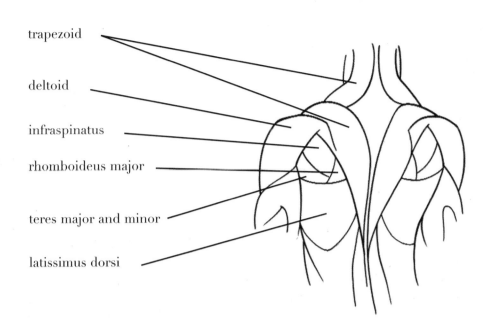

trapezoid

deltoid

infraspinatus

rhomboideus major

teres major and minor

latissimus dorsi

Right:
The muscles of the back change quite dramatically when the arms are raised. At the sides the latissimus dorsi and serratus muscles gain prominence while the two sections of the trapezius are brought closer towards the shoulder, causing a deepening of the gulley between them

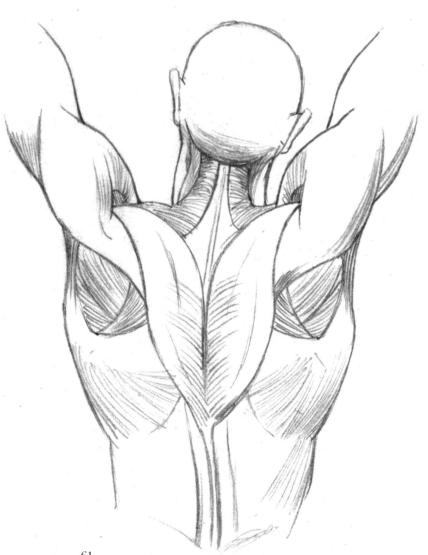

THE SHOULDER

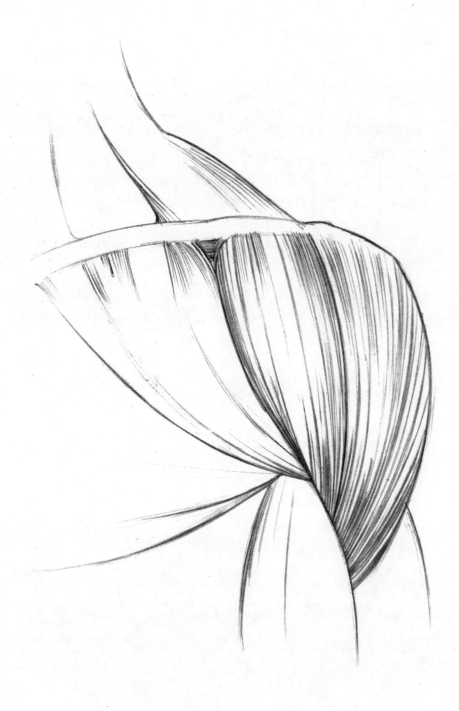

The shoulder is composed of the powerful *deltoid* muscle which lays over the shoulder joint. It is attached to the lateral third of the clavicle as seen at left, as well as at the scapula at both its spine and acromion. From here it moves downwards to it's insertion point about one-third of the way down on the lateral shaft of the humerus at the deltoid tuberosity. See page 16 for a detailed image of this.

The principle action of the deltoid is in lifting the arm. As it is a multipennate muscle - one mass, but sectioned - the shape of the deltoid alters dependant on the position of the arm and the action performed.

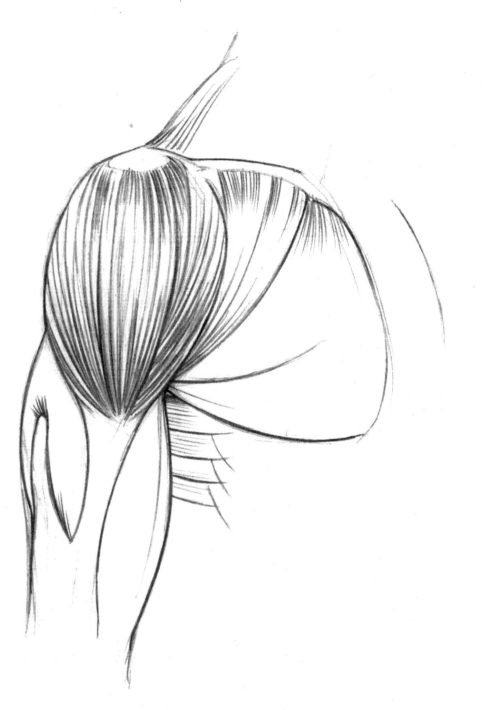

In this oblique lateral view of the deltoid we can see more clearly the origin and insertion points as well as its proximity to the bicep and tricep muscles. Notice that the scapula at the very top of the shoulder is covered with only a thin layer of ligament and skin. This is the point where the trapezius is rooted, as described on the following page.

scapula

deltoid

pectoralis major - clavicular part

tricep

bicep

SHOULDER MOVEMENT

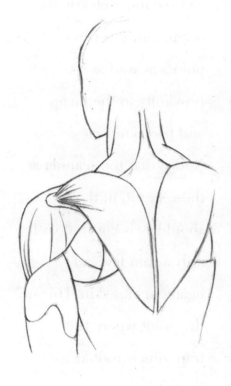

This set of drawings clearly shows the movement of the muscles at the shoulder as the arm is raised. The important point to note is that the trapezius muscle is firmly rooted at the scapula and does not rise with the deltoid. Instead, a divot is formed by the movement of the deltoid as the arm moves through its arc until the arm is fully extended upwards.

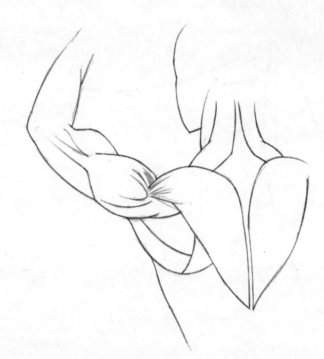

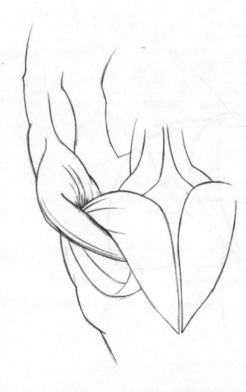

Getting this wrong is one of the commonest mistakes made by the novice. Due to the unique structure of the shoulder, assumptions we might make about it prove to be false.

For this reason, it can be one of the epiphanous moments in our understanding of anatomy. The whole shoulder area, from the acromion to the armpit is one of the most troublesome there is: we need to give it plenty of study.

THE FRONT

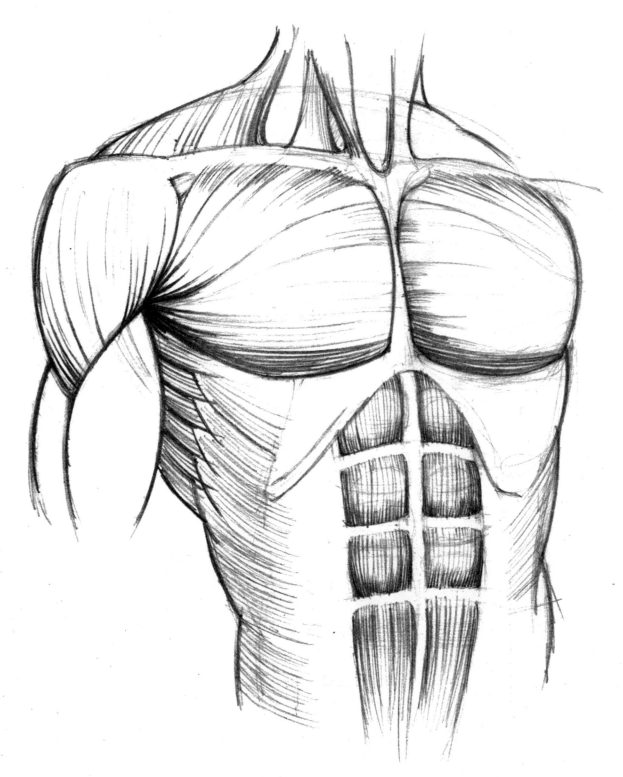

Two areas of muscle dominate the front of the torso: the *pectoralis* muscles and the *rectus abdominis* group, more commonly referred to as abdominal muscles or 'abs'. The abdominals tend to protrude only on very lean people such as athletes. They run from the pubic region and widen as they move up towards their attachment point at the costal cartilages of the ribs.

THE PECTORALS

The *pectoralis major* muscle of the chest originates over a very wide area: from the clavicle, adjacent to the deltoid, along the length of the clavicle, then along about half of the sternum and onto the costal cartilages of the true ribs. Their insertion point is, after a tight twisting and flattening of the tendon, into the upper part of the humerus. Pectoralis major is composed of two sections: the clavicular part, which as the name suggests is that section attached to the collar bone. The other section is fittingly named the sternocostal part. The purpose of this large muscle is to move the arm across the body. It's used when we grip things tightly to our bodies and when we mold or crush things in our hands.

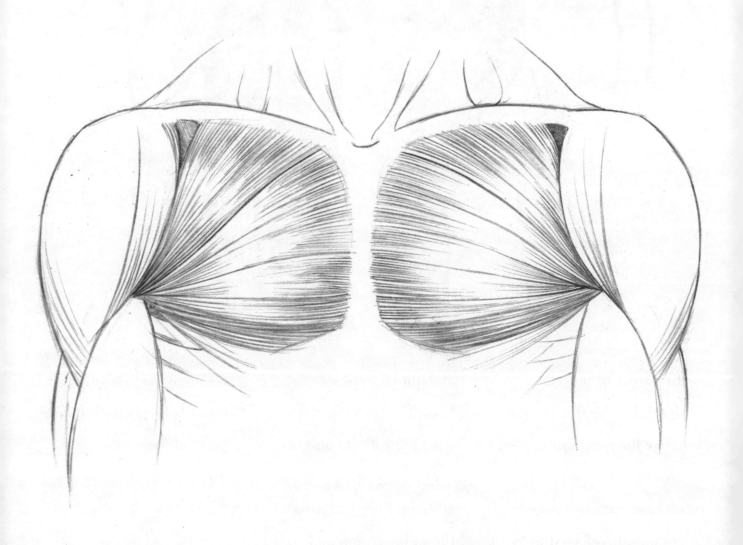

The *pectoralis minor* muscle is almost entirely covered by the huge mass of its larger relation. the only section of it ever likely to be seen by the artist is a small triangular section forming part of the underarm.

At right is a side view of pectoralis major showing the twisting of the muscle as it forms the tendon.

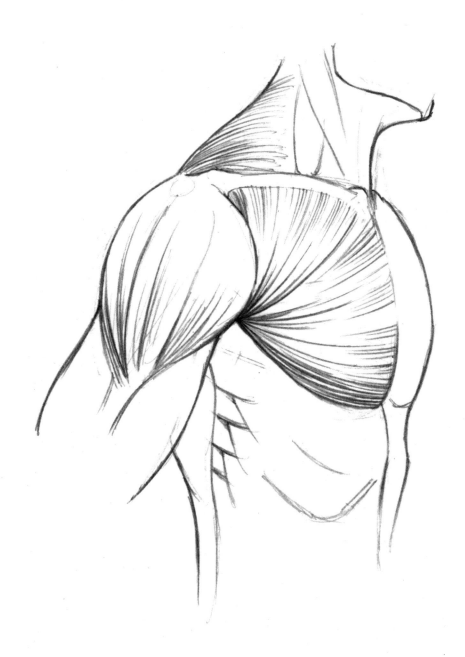

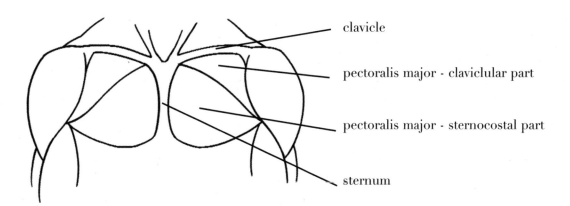

clavicle

pectoralis major - claviclular part

pectoralis major - sternocostal part

sternum

MOVING PARTS

As is illustrated in the images on these two pages, the shape of the muscles of the torso can be highly changeable, depending on posture. When the arms are raised, the pectorals can alter their appearance quite dramatically. This should come as no great surprise as they are attached to so much of the upper body.

Studying the movements of athletes is an excellent way of gathering information about the interaction of muscle groups. There's an endless amount of material in magazines or on the internet. The challenge of correctly identifying the muscles even when they are in a highly unconventional position can only be of benefit.

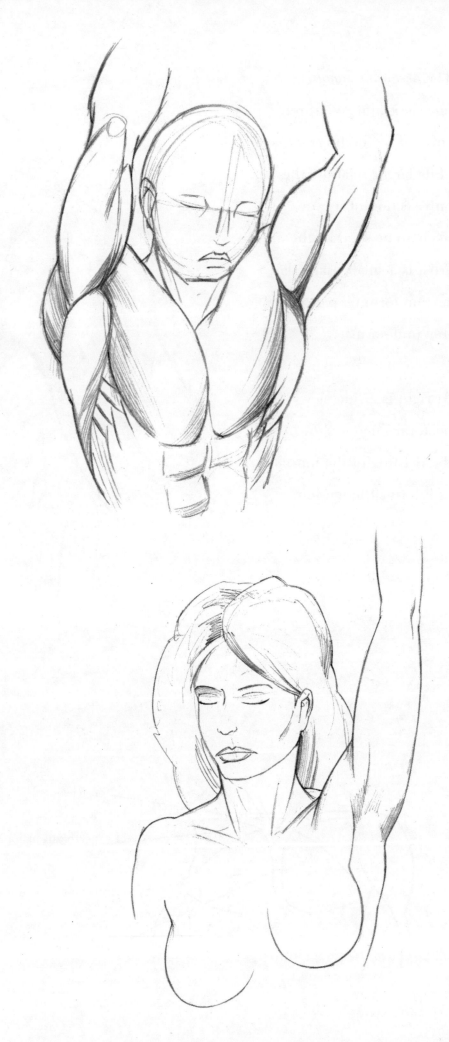

As the abdominal muscles do not lie across bone but rather are free floating, they will stretch or compress in inverse relationship to the movement of the spine. As the torso twists, so will the abdominals. Another good way of getting the information into our heads is to continuously draw only one area. Two days of concentrated drawing on the upper back may at first sound like a tedious prospect, but may well lead to a breakthrough in our understanding.

As we study the workings of the body, we usually end up becoming more aware of the functions of our own anatomy. This in turn gives us a better 'feel' for the subject, as our understanding of what is in front of us becomes more instinctual and less intellectual. I believe drawing is at its best when the whole of the person holding the pencil is engaged, mind *and* body.

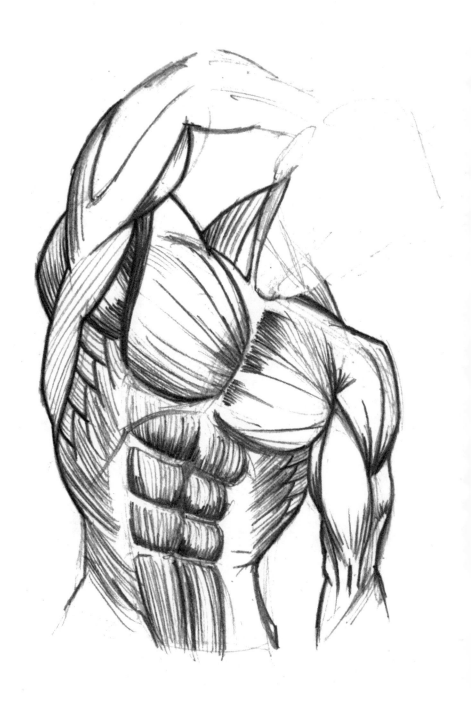

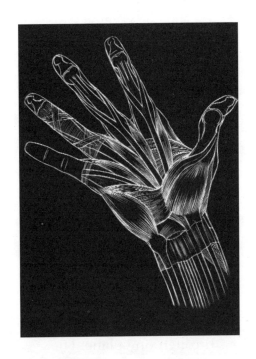

ARM & HAND

THE ARM
PART 1: THE BONES

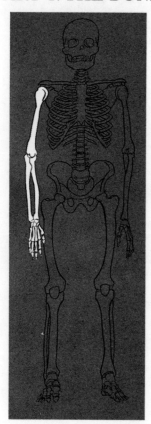

Three bones make up the human arm: the upper arm has just one bone, the *humerus*. The forearm is composed of two bones, the *radius* and *ulna*. The humerus is approximately one-fifth of the body's total length, second in length only to the femur (upper leg bone).

The humerus and scapula join at the shoulder in what is known as a synovial joint. These joints typically allow a large degree of articulation and their points of contact are covered with hyaline cartilage, an ultra-smooth surface which eliminates friction between the moving parts. These joints also have synovial membranes lining the joint which secrete synovial fluid, ensuring the surface of the joint is properly lubricated.

The elbow joint is a somewhat different arrangement, as it only allows for movement through one plane. The elbow is a synovial hinge joint and its single plane articulation is accounted for by the very shape of the joint between the humerus and ulna. This shape makes free rotation of the joint impossible.

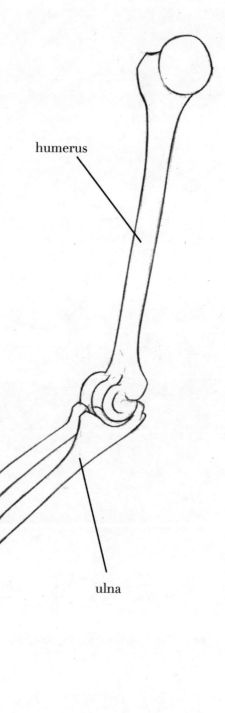

humerus

radius

ulna

UPPER ARM BONE: THE HUMERUS

The humerus can be broken down into three main sections.

The head contains the hemispherical protrusion seen at the top of the bone. This is the part which connects to the shoulder joint.

The shaft makes up most of the length of the bone. On its surface are ridges and grooves which serve to aid the attachment of ligaments. The shaft terminates in a collection of notches and shapes, all with a very specific purpose. These form one-half of the hinge mechanism by which the elbow articulates.

At right is a posterior view of the left humerus. At bottom left we can see a round protrusion called the *capitulum*. This is the part of the humerus that the radius is married up to. At bottom right is the *trochlea*, which marries up with the head of the ulna.

At the far left is a protrusion called the *medial epicondyle*, better known to most people as the funny bone. Between a third and halfway down is a bump called the *deltoid tuberosity*. This is the insert point for the large shoulder muscle.

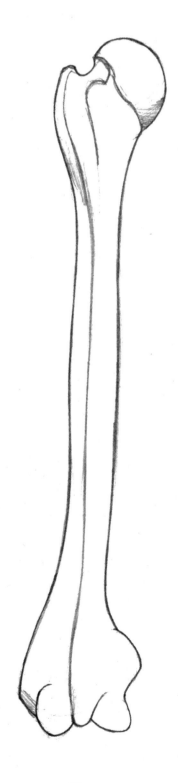

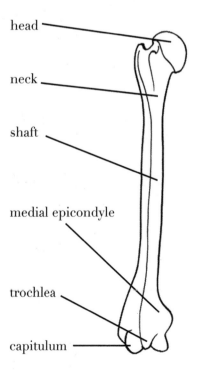

head

neck

shaft

medial epicondyle

trochlea

capitulum

RADIUS AND ULNA

The skeleton of the lower arm is made up of two bones; the *radius* and the *ulna*.

The radius is connected to the humerus at the capitulum by the head of the radius.

The ulna is connected at the trochlea of the humerus by the coronoid process of the ulna.

The trochlea in particular, together with the coronoid process is the restricting part of the elbow. When an arm is straightened at the elbow the coronoid process and trochlea effectively lock the joint, preventing further movement.

One obvious feature of these two arm bones is the fact that they both taper, but in different directions. Remembering that it's the ulna that is broadest at the elbow can help us a lot when making figure drawing decisions.

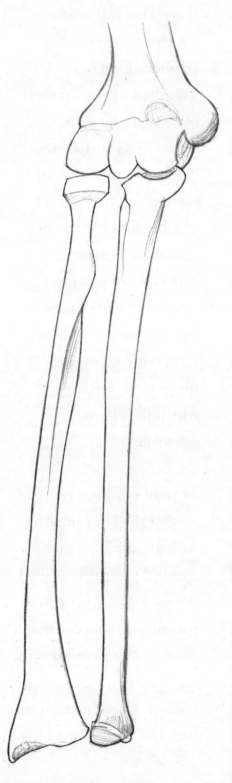

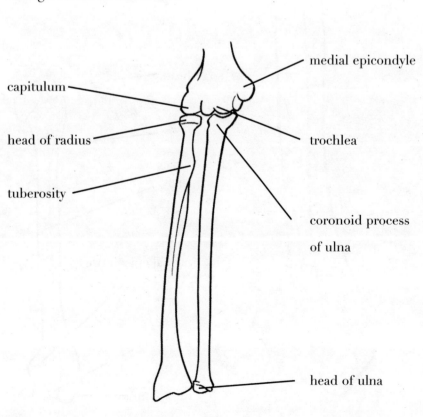

capitulum

medial epicondyle

head of radius

trochlea

tuberosity

coronoid process of ulna

head of ulna

SHOULDER JOINT

The head of the humerus fits snugly into the shoulder at the *glenoid process*. The joint is then held in tightly by an arrangement of ligaments attached to both the *acromion* and the *coracoid process*, parts of the clavicle or shoulder blade, as een on page 17.

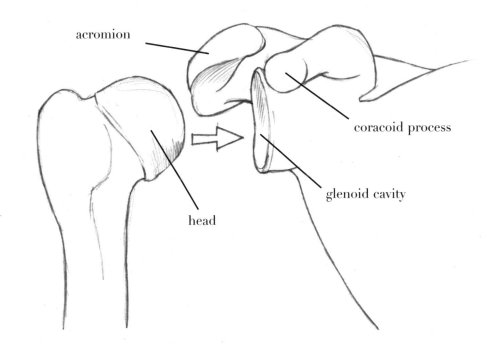

acromion

coracoid process

glenoid cavity

head

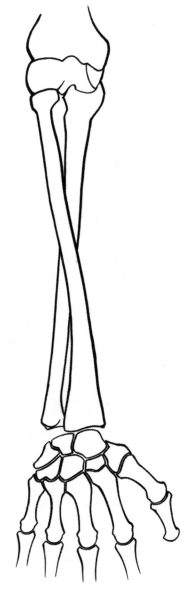

WRIST ACTION

At left is a demonstration of why a two bone arrangement, rather than a swivel-type joint is a good idea. When we rotate our wrist, the radius and ulna allow us approximately 180 degrees of movement. Unlike the swivel arrangement of the shoulder, the elbow only allows movement in one direction. In combination with the much freer shoulder joint, we can achieve all the articulation we need for any task.

PART 2:
THE MUSCLES

Although the deltoid muscles form part of their shoulders, they are intimately connected with the muscles of the upper arm. The biceps in particular seem to flow out of the deltoids, so any consideration of the muscles of the upper arm has to begin with a consideration of the relationship between these two muscle groups.

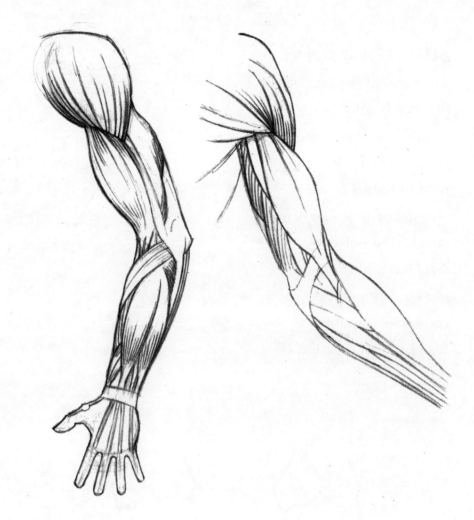

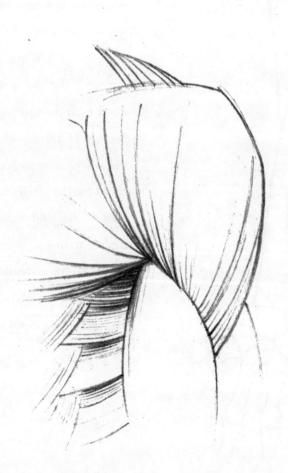

The muscle area shown at left is among the most complicated in the human body. It is a point where several different muscle groups all converge. If we can fully understand how all of these groups interact, our understanding of anatomy as a whole will be hugely improved.

In this drawing you should be able to identify the *pectoral*, *deltoid*, *bicep*, *tricep* and *serratus* muscles.

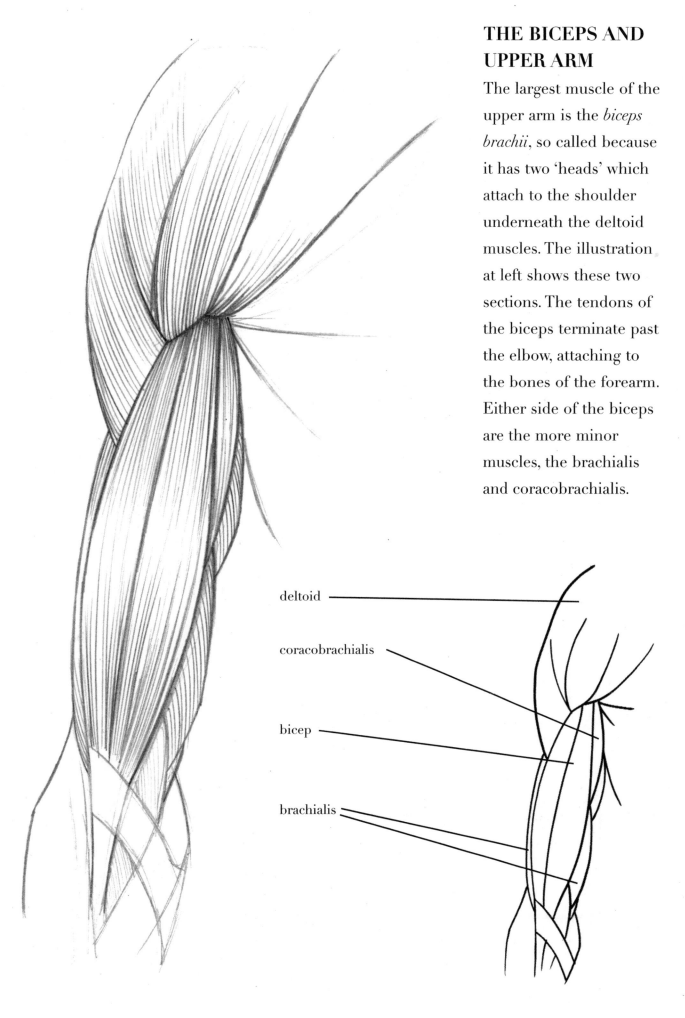

THE BICEPS AND UPPER ARM

The largest muscle of the upper arm is the *biceps brachii*, so called because it has two 'heads' which attach to the shoulder underneath the deltoid muscles. The illustration at left shows these two sections. The tendons of the biceps terminate past the elbow, attaching to the bones of the forearm. Either side of the biceps are the more minor muscles, the brachialis and coracobrachialis.

deltoid

coracobrachialis

bicep

brachialis

TRICEPS MUSCLES

These muscles have three
'heads', thus the name
triceps. As with the
biceps these heads are
buried under the
deltoids.

The tendon of the lateral
head emanate from the
back of the humerus. The
long head tendon from
the shoulder joint.

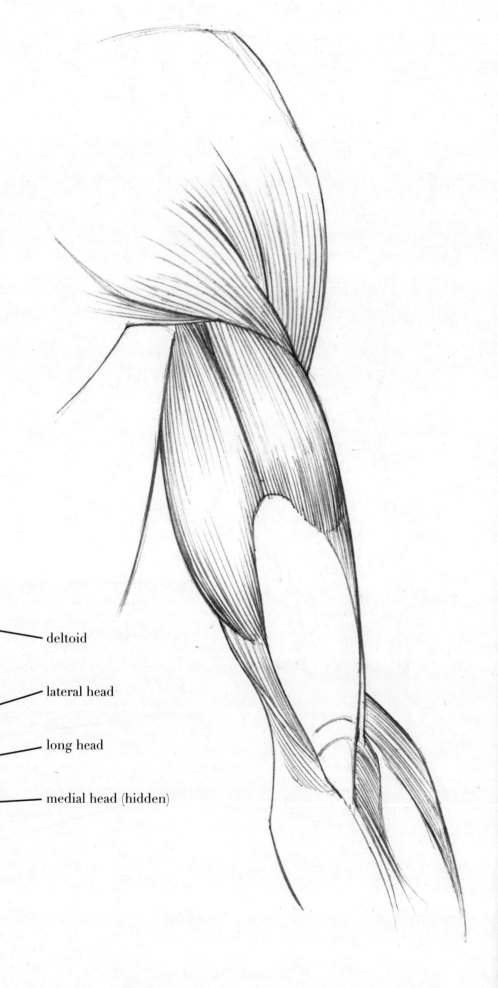

deltoid

lateral head

long head

medial head (hidden)

UP OR DOWN?

These two drawings illustrate the major differences in function of the triceps and biceps muscles. The biceps are classic *flexor* muscles, the triceps are *extensors*. Flexors bend, extensors straighten.

Drawing A shows an arm exercising downward force, for instance pulling on a rope. The triceps can perform this particular function with no help at all from the biceps.

If the same arm in the same position exercises upward force i.e. bending the limb, it is the biceps which perform the work. Again, the triceps need play no part in this action.

These considerations are important when figure drawing as large muscle groups are very eloquent indicators of the kind of action a body is involved in. Stress the wrong muscles and our figures will look stiff, confusing or just plain wrong.

A

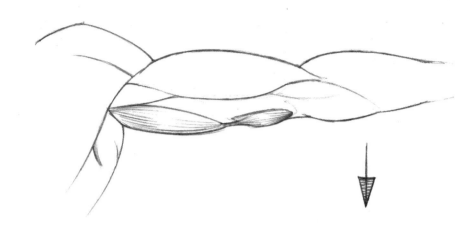

B

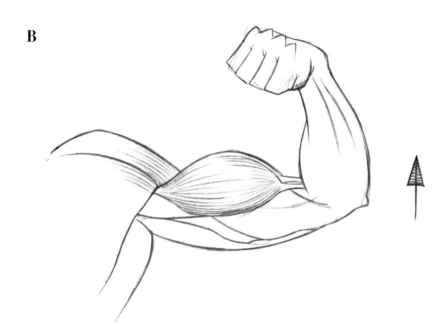

Drawing B above also demonstrates exactly how a contracting muscle exerts force on the lower part of the limb, pulling it upward. The more weight the forearm is carrying, the more extreme the contraction of the bicep will be. Just about everybody, non-artists included, knows that the way to show that great effort is being exerted is to push the contraction of these muscles to their limits.

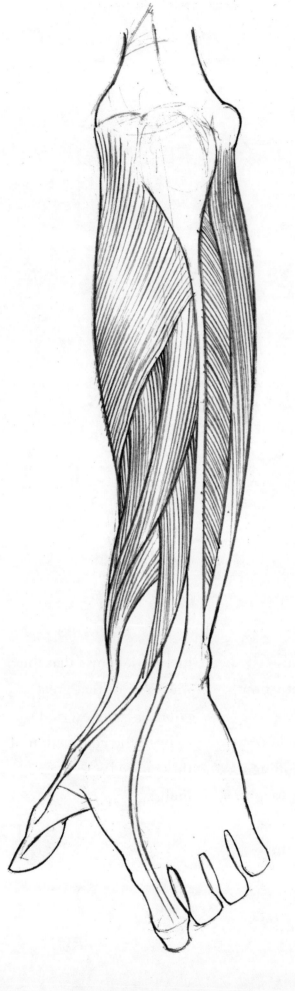

Because the muscles are built up over the skeleton in layers, they are usually illustrated in medical anatomy books as a series of levels.

Although the artist is primarily concerned with the surface of the human body, no proper understanding of the surface can be reached without some knowledge of the way in which these layers are built up.

The first layer, that is the layer which is in

supinator

flexor carpi ulnaris

abductor pollicis longus

extensor pollicis brevis

abductor pollicis longus

immediate contact with the skeleton is known as the *deep layer*. The deep layer of the forearm is shown here at left.

To an extent, this division into layers is arbitrary, as muscles tend to weave above and below each other. However, it is a useful way of bringing clarity to a complex arrangement of muscles and tendons, particularly in this case where there are a large number of components to deal with.

The illustration on this page shows the *superficial layer* of the forearm.

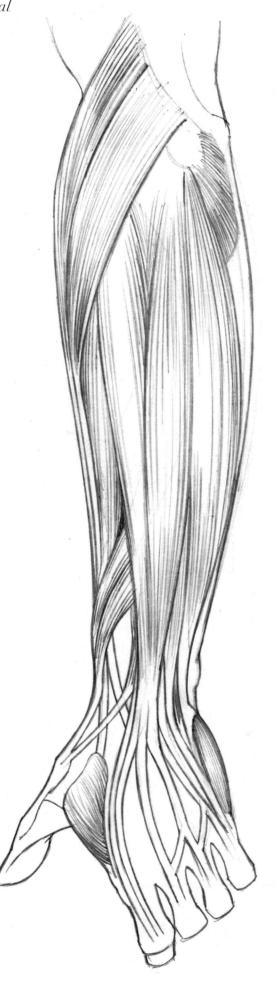

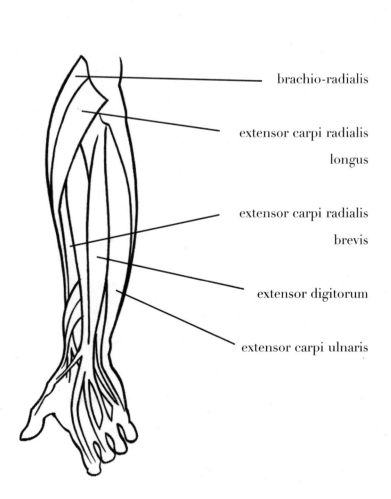

brachio-radialis

extensor carpi radialis longus

extensor carpi radialis brevis

extensor digitorum

extensor carpi ulnaris

In this view of the forearm the most prominent muscle is the *brachio-radialis*. The other muscles originate at the medial epicondyle (see page 65) and with the exception of *pronator teres* flow into the wrist as tendons.

Flexor carpi radialis and *flexor carpi ulnaris* attach at the metacarpal bones (see next page) and are used for wrist movement.

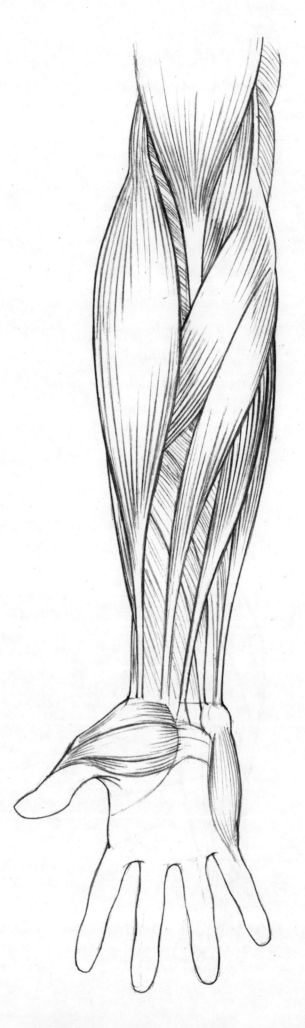

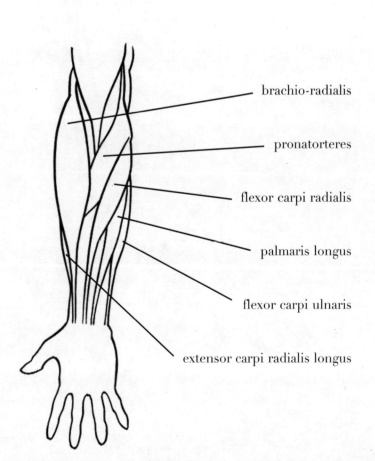

brachio-radialis

pronatorteres

flexor carpi radialis

palmaris longus

flexor carpi ulnaris

extensor carpi radialis longus

THE HAND
PART 1: THE BONES

If we were to ask an artist early in their learning what was giving them the most difficulty, chances are they'd reply "hands". A quick glance at the drawing at right gives us some idea why.

The human hand has a high concentration of small bones in a very compact area. It is also the most adaptable area of the body, capable of a very wide range of movements. For these reasons, it's a good idea to take our time when learning about the skeletal, muscular and superficial aspects of the hand.

The bones of the fingers are called *phalanges*. Each phalanx, from knuckle to fingertip successively reduces in size by almost one-half. The large bones which make up the palm are called *metacarpals*. Seven loosely interlocking bones called

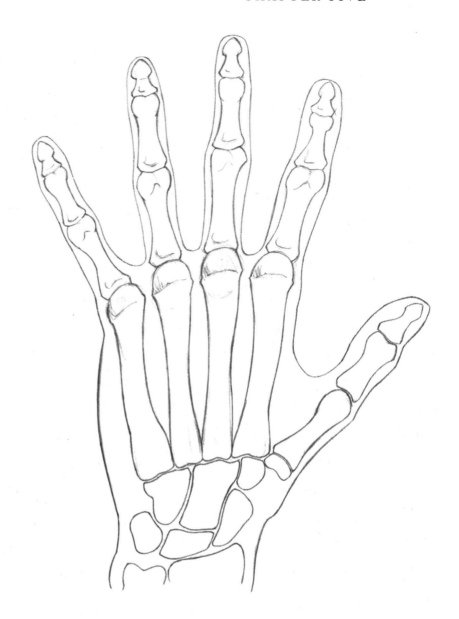

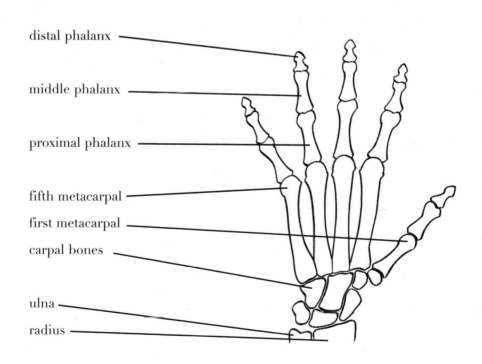

distal phalanx

middle phalanx

proximal phalanx

fifth metacarpal

first metacarpal

carpal bones

ulna

radius

83

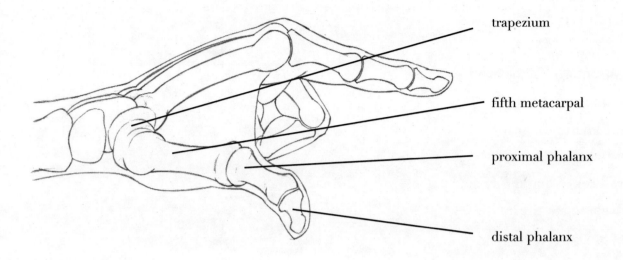

trapezium

fifth metacarpal

proximal phalanx

distal phalanx

the carpal bones make up the wrist section.
The joints between the metacarpals and the phalanges are of the ball-and-socket type, allowing a large degree of freedom. However, the joints between phalanges are of a rocker type, allowing movement through only one plane. The thumb has only two

phalanges and is joined to the wrist where a carpal bone called the *trapezium* meets the fifth metacarpal. Its freedom

of movement is restricted only by the triangle of muscle and skin between the thumb and forefinger.

Right:

cross-section of the bones of one finger. Held in place by tendons and flexor sheaths, the concave bases of the phalanges are able to move across the convex heads of the phalanx beneath through one plane of movement only.

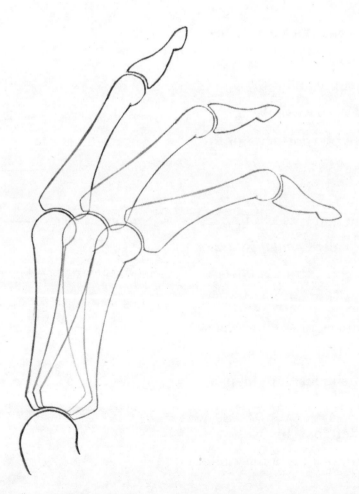

THE HAND
PART 2:
THE MUSCLES

The sheer number of tendons terminating in the hand can make learning the workings of the hand a daunting task. The illustrations on this and the next page have simplified the components to those that are essential to our understanding.

As the tendons of the flexor and extensor muscles of the forearm pass into the wrist, they do so beneath bands of fibres called *retinaculae*. These bands make sure the tendons remain in their positions as the muscles are flexed or extended.

The tendons will become prominent, particularly on the back of the hand, when their muscles of origin are brought into use. In the case of those illustrated at right, those leading to the fingers on the dorsal side of the hand belong to the

extensor digitorum muscle, buried deep in the forearm.
The two prominent

tendons leading to the base of the thumb are of the extensor muscles *pollicis brevis* and *pollicis longus*.

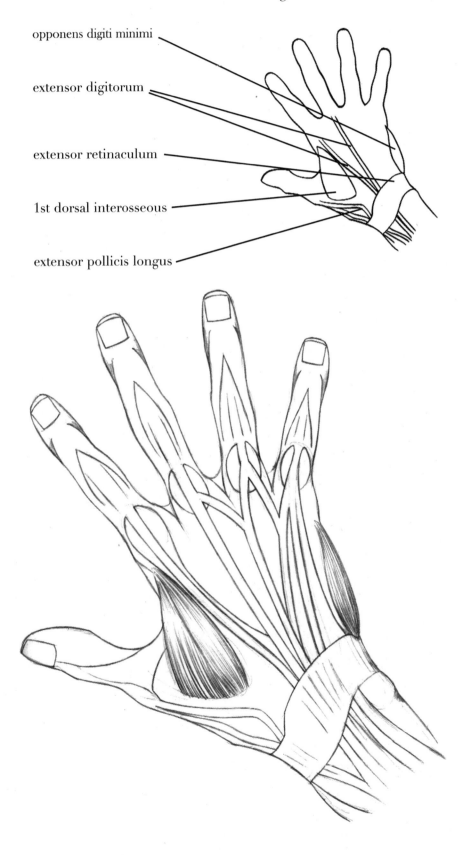

opponens digiti minimi

extensor digitorum

extensor retinaculum

1st dorsal interosseous

extensor pollicis longus

THE PALM

The bulk of the muscle mass of the hand is found at the palm. Of particular prominence is the large area known as the *thenar eminence* or base of the thumb. This area is composed of three muscles: *flexor pollicis brevis*, *abductor pollicis brevis* and *opponens pollicis*, the key muscles involved in thumb movement.

On the medial side of the palm are the *hypothenar* muscles, responsible for the abduction and flexing of the little finger. *Abductor digiti minimi* and *flexor digiti minimi* can for the purposes of drawing be treated as one muscle. To the right of these lies the third of the hypothenar muscles, *opponens digiti minimi*. Bridging the thenar and hypothenar muscles is the *palmaris brevis*. Running alongside each of the *flexor digitorum* tendons are the *lumbrical muscles*. These have the specific job of flexing the

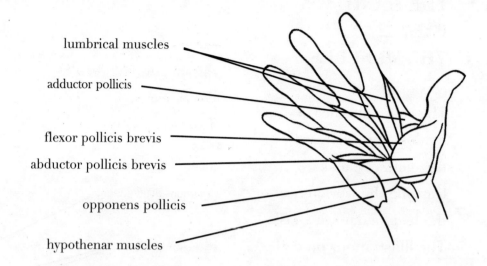

lumbrical muscles

adductor pollicis

flexor pollicis brevis

abductor pollicis brevis

opponens pollicis

hypothenar muscles

joint between the metacarpals and the proximal palanges. If you've forgotten where these are, see page 83. As with elsewhere on the wrist and hands, sheaths of thin, tough fibre bind the many tendons of the digits in place, helping to create a highly compact, versatile and strong package.

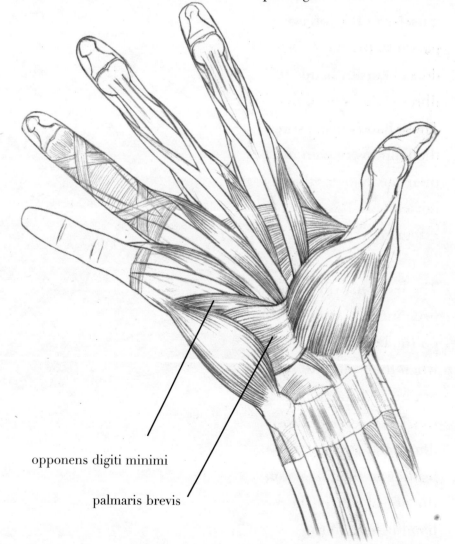

opponens digiti minimi

palmaris brevis

86

REAL HANDS

We've just covered a lot of information regarding the workings of the hand. Now let's put some of that information to practical use.

When drawing any part of the anatomy from life we should first and foremost look at what is in front of us. This means not to prejudge or draw what we think is there, and certainly not what our imaginations think should be there. Drawing from life means not allowing our imaginations to influence the outcome.

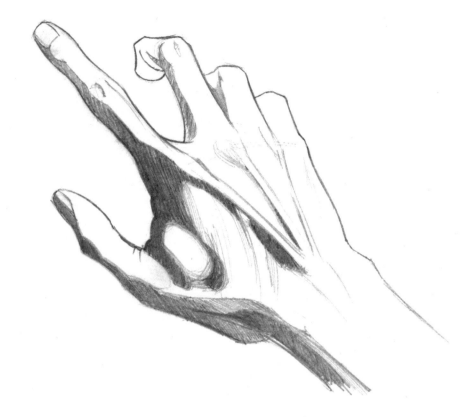

There is , however, a legitimate part of our mental process we can use. Knowledge of the workings of the body will help ensure that what we draw is convincing, that what the viewer sees is a functional example of a part of human anatomy that they themselves also possess.

This is part of what makes anatomy the greatest challenge. Everyone has an instinctive grasp of any drawing's believability, as they themselves possess a working example of the thing being drawn.

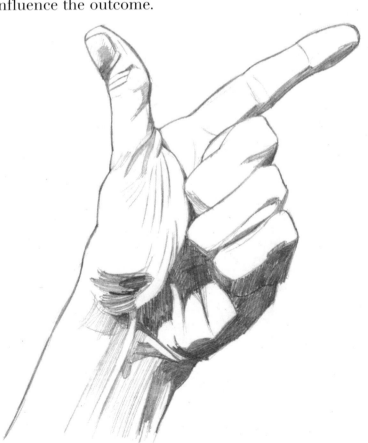

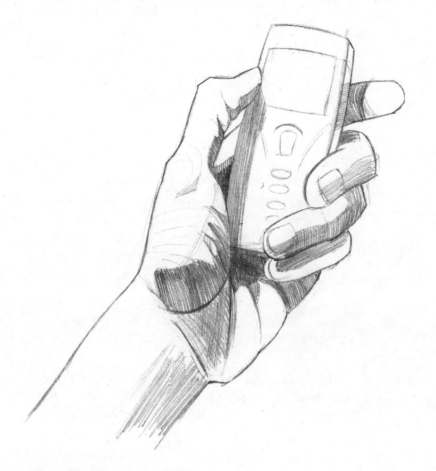

comes into contact with the flesh of the hand. What effects does the much harder surface of the phone have on the soft flesh?

positioning of the digits: the thumb and fingers have to work in unison to form a convincing grip. This is especially true in the case of the image below. A hand holding a pencil involves a wide variety of angles. The pencil rests on the third and fourth fingers, but is gripped by the first and second in conjunction with the thumb. The pencil is also stabilized at the fold between thumb and forefinger.

GRIPPING

Hands interacting with tools presents us with one of the more difficult challenges. Achieving a high degree of naturalism in this discipline can be highly satisfying. Things to be aware of can include the following:

points of contact: to get the mobile phone in the image above to rest loosely but comfortably in the grip of the hand requires careful observation. Pay particularly close attention to the exact points where the phone

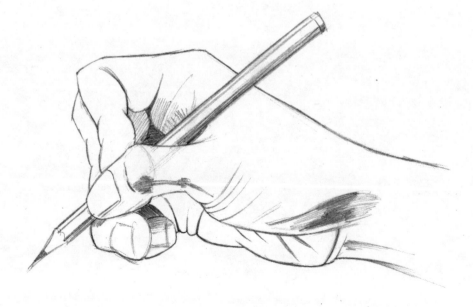

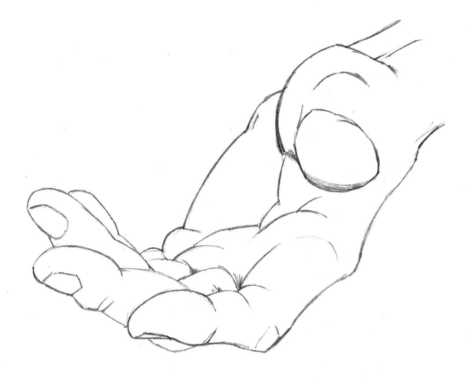

as shown in the drawing at right, these sections become more convex. The way these parts of the digits and palm interact can be extremely subtle and difficult to master. The more studies we produce, the closer we will be to building up a complete three-dimensional 'map' of the hands in our heads. We can then use this map to enable us to make the right decisions about what to include and what to leave out, as ultimately these decisions are what really guides the viewer into making sense of what they see.

FOLDS OF SKIN

Another key aspect of drawing the hand is understanding how the various sections of skin behave as the hand changes shape or position.

In the above drawing the hand is neither flexed or extended, representing a relaxed position. We can clearly see the slightly convex shapes of the skin covering the fingers. If the fingers are extended, we know that these will flatten out. Likewise if we draw the fingers inward

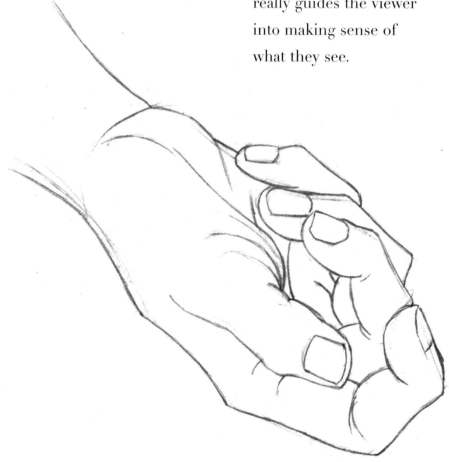

PLANNING

Sometimes we can set ourselves a drawing task so complex that we have little chance of it coming out right unless we begin with an overall plan of what we want to achieve. A typical example of this is the pair of loosely interlocking hands on these pages.

1: Block out the positions of the palms first, remembering that one has to be higher than the other. Next, we need to indicate the lines along

1

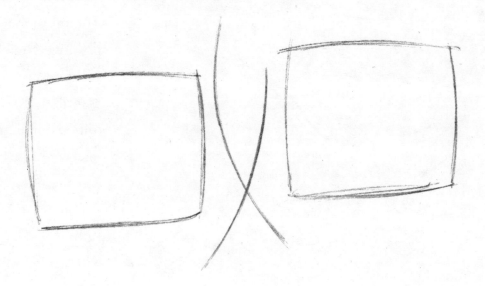

which both sets of knuckles lie.
2: Use the lines just drawn to indicate the positions of the knuckles of both hands. Pay

particular attention at the point where the third fingers intersect. The knuckles should be roughly equidistant but diminishing in size as

they move down the lines.
3: Now we need to fit the fingers between each other, add the wrists and thumbs and give the palms their shape.

2

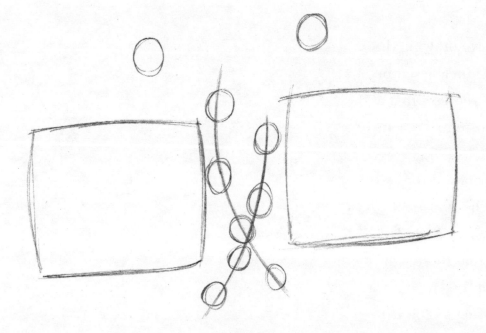

3

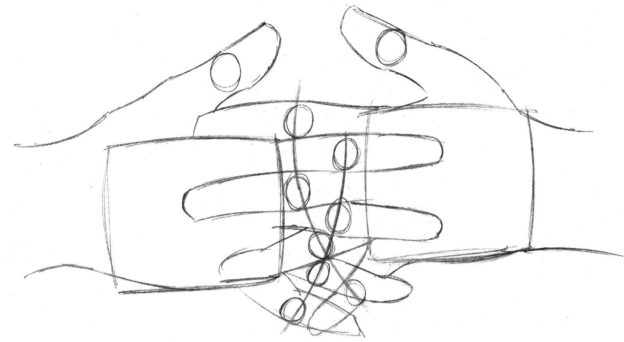

As a guide, remember that the forefingers should reach to just beyond the point where the thumb meets the palm. Notice also that the tips of the fingers follow the same arc pattern as the lines for drawing 1.

4: Before putting in the details and light you'll want to erase your original guidelines. Hopefully, you'll be left with a clean framework on which to finish your drawing.

Planning of this kind is all about pattern recognition - seeing past the superficial and into what lies beneath. Most seemingly complex structures, provided they are not completely random can have this approach applied to them, giving us the confidence that the finished drawing will be structurally sound.

4

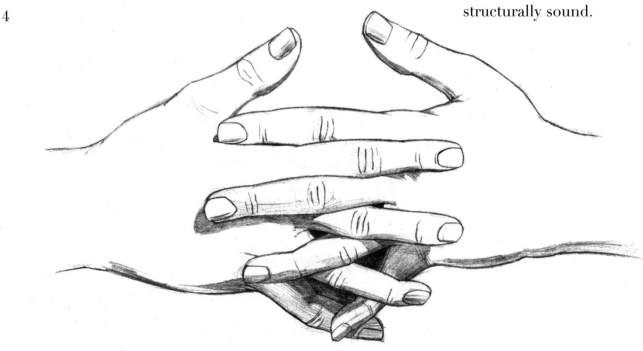

The drawing at right has
been done without
toning. It is a deliberately
unsubtle study of the
digits and their joints
when used for holding,
cradling etc.

More subtle is the study
of working hands below.
The object is to show the
relationship between two
hands involved in a
shared task.

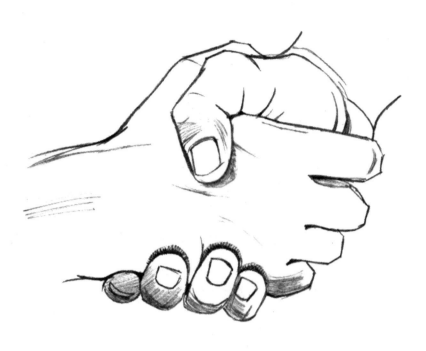

The handshake is an excellent subject for helping us to understand the dynamics of the human hand. How does a loose grip differ from a firm one? Why does the third finger project further forward than the longer second finger? The way in which two hands lock in a handshake speaks volumes about the hand's design. Try studying this from several different angles.

Below is a classic human action - the point. With the forefinger coming straight at us, the foreshortening is intense. We need to really study the joints of the forefinger in order to get this to work. Equally as important are the stressed areas of skin coming down from the knuckle. If the viewer doesn't 'get' the foreshortened finger alone, these folds of skin act as a signifier for what is being portrayed.

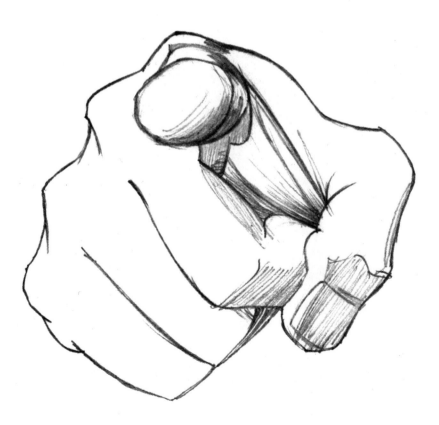

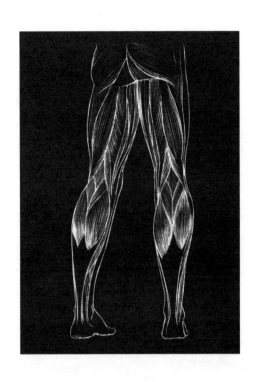

LEG AND FOOT

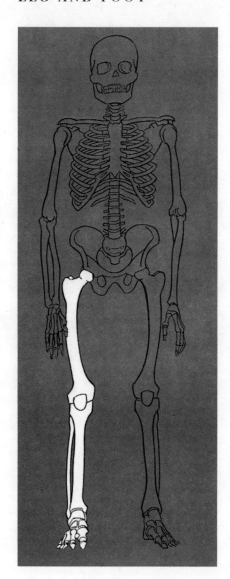

BONES OF THE LEG

The Femur

The *femur*, or thigh bone is the longest bone in the human body. It is usually at least one quarter of the body's total length. It has three main sections; the head, the shaft and terminates in one half of the hinge joint that forms the knee, the largest joint in the body. The two large, rounded sections at the base of the femur are known as *condyles*. The protrusions emanating from below the neck of the femur are the greater and lesser trochanters. In life the greater trochanter is highly prominent, especially in females.

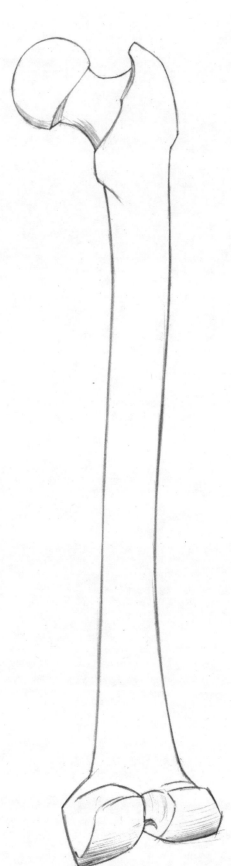

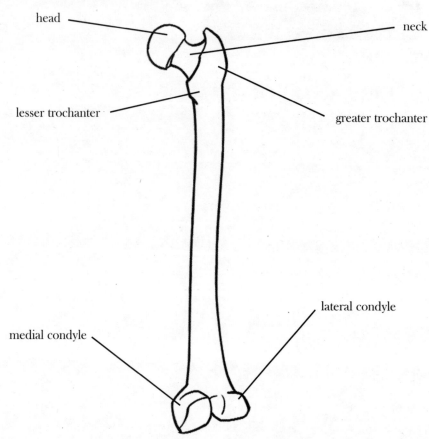

head

neck

lesser trochanter

greater trochanter

lateral condyle

medial condyle

THE HIP JOINT

The head of the femur is attached to the pelvis by insertion into a socket type indentation known as the *acetabulum* (see pages 56 & 57). This allows the femur to move very freely in near-unlimited articulation. As with the humerus and shoulder, it is a synovial type joint; a highly smooth surface which is continually lubricated by synovial fluid. As with the shoulder joint, the hip joint is encapsulated by ligaments.

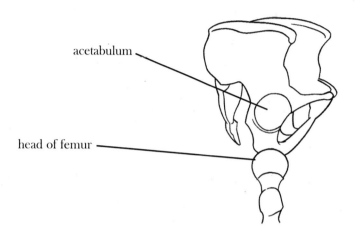

acetabulum

head of femur

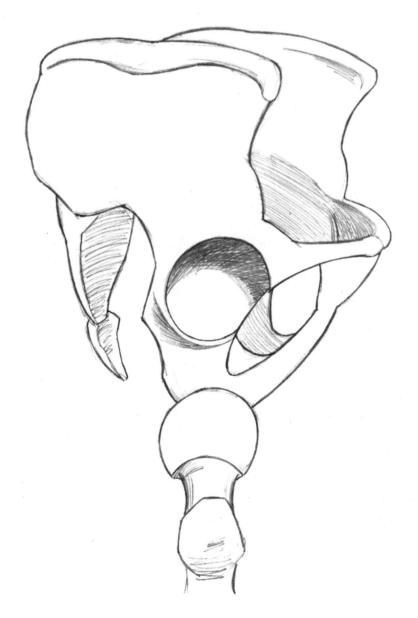

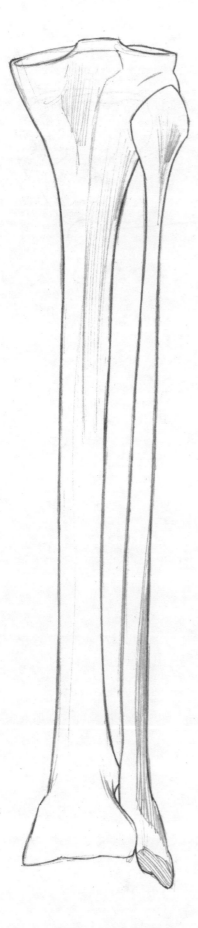

Tibia and Fibula

As is obvious in the illustration on this page, the bones of the lower leg differ greatly in size. The larger of the two is the tibia, being the sole supporter of weight and the part that makes up the lower half of the knee joint.

The fibula is more closely associated with the articulation of the ankle but also provides mooring for important muscles as we shall see later.

This illustration shows a front view of the left leg and it should be easy to recognize some of the features which lie very close to the surface of the skin. The head of the fibula tends to show as a small protrusion at the outside of the knee joint. It should also be obvious that the ankle is in fact two bones. If you really want to know, each of these parts where the bones form the ankle is known as a *malleolus*.

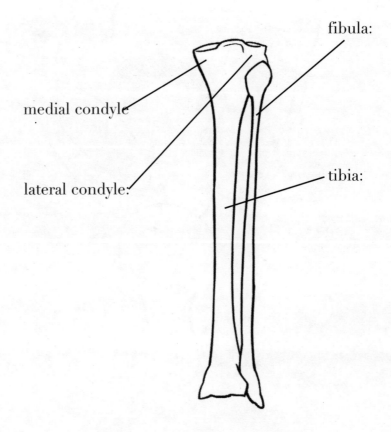

fibula:

medial condyle

lateral condyle:

tibia:

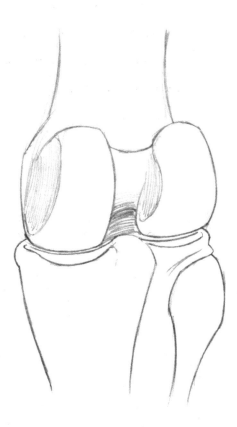

Knee Joint
The illustration at left shows a rear view of the right knee joint. The condyles of the joint are plain to see. The condyles of the femur are free to rock back and forth over those of the tibia. We can also see from this that the knee joint is designed strictly to bend in one direction only - the perfectly rounded parts of the condyle are situated at the back of the knee only.

Knee Joint - front
There are actually two joints at the front of the knee. The first, between the Femur and Tibia is discussed above. The second is between the *patella*, or knee cap and the femur. The patella is attached at its top to the quadriceps muscle of the thigh and at the bottom to the tibial tubercle. When the quadriceps are contracted, this pulls on the patella which in turn lifts the tibia. There is a notch at the base of the femur called the trochlear groove which allows the patella to perform this important function.

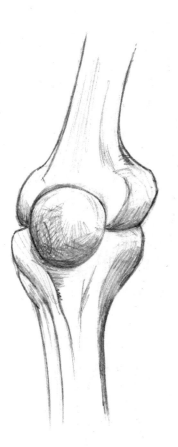

Muscles of the Leg
1: The thigh
The muscles of the human leg can be particularly perplexing for those starting to get to grips with anatomy. Fortunately, there are ways in which we can make our life easier. The long, strap-like muscle running diagonally from the hip to the inside of the knee is called the *sartorius*. If we can correctly place this muscle it can be an immense help in mapping out the rest of the leg muscles. The large *rectus femoris* flows out of the knee and up at a slight angle, widening as it does, until it reaches the point between the sartorius and *tensor fasciae latae*. The muscles of the inner thigh tend to be overshadowed by

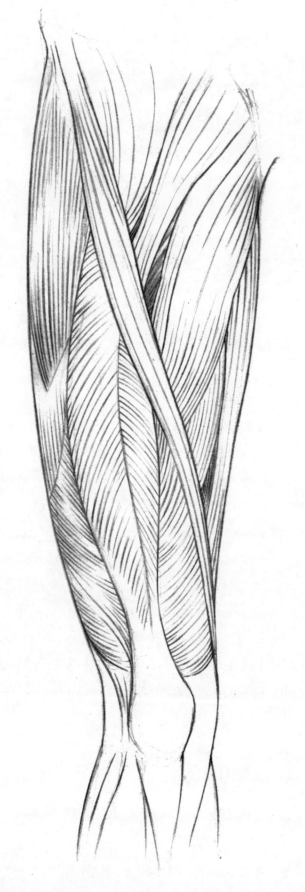

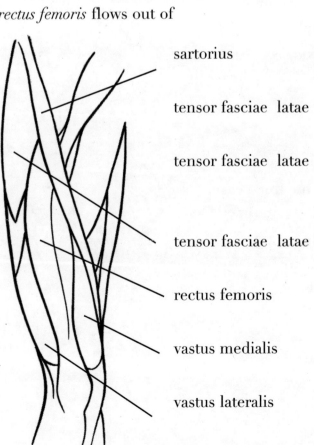

sartorius

tensor fasciae latae

tensor fasciae latae

tensor fasciae latae

rectus femoris

vastus medialis

vastus lateralis

those just mentioned, due to their much lesser degree of protrusion at the surface.

The side of the thigh is a little less complex and includes the most massive muscle in the body, the

gluteus maximus. Running from the outside of the knee to the *gluteus medius* is a sheath-like covering called the *iliotibial tract*. We can also see the vastus lateralis from the previous page, along with the rectus femoris in front of it.

At the rear of the thigh is the *biceps femoris* which attaches at the outside of the knee with a tendon often clearly visible in reality.

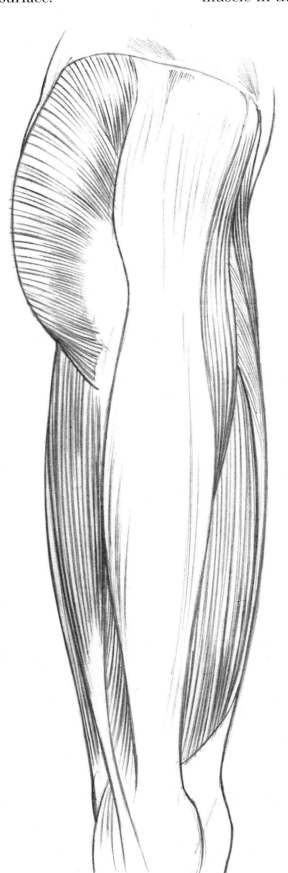

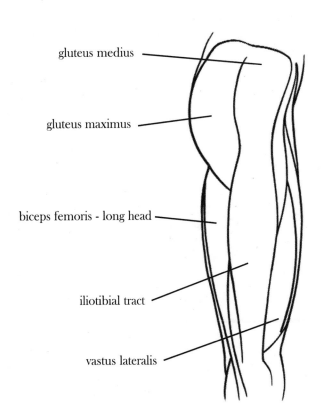

gluteus medius

gluteus maximus

biceps femoris - long head

iliotibial tract

vastus lateralis

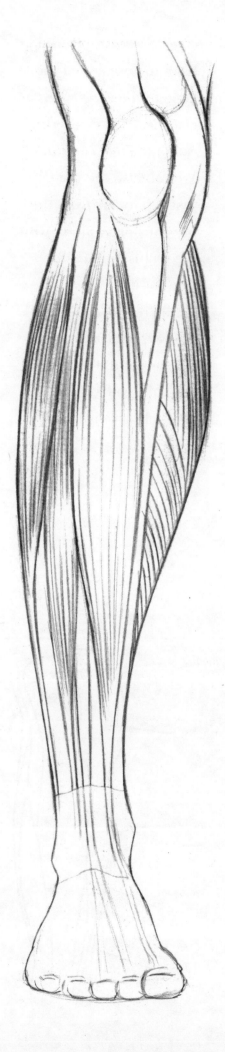

2: The Lower Leg

As we did with the thigh, we should try to locate key muscles of the lower leg to help orient ourselves. The most obvious muscle at first glance is the *tibialis anterior*. This muscle runs at a gentle diagonal from the outside of the knee, specifically from the lateral condyle, down to the inside of the foot, eventually joining at the first metatarsal bone. Flex this muscle and you will clearly see its tendon between your ankles.

Next to the tibialis anterior, on the lateral side, is another extensor muscle, the *peroneus longus*. Between the two is its partner *peroneus brevis*. They're primarily concerned with turning the feet. Try this yourself, and again, you should clearly be able to feel them, especially if you turn your foot upwards. On the medial side, we can see part of the mighty *gastrocnemius*, the most powerful of the lower leg muscles and better known as the calf muscles.

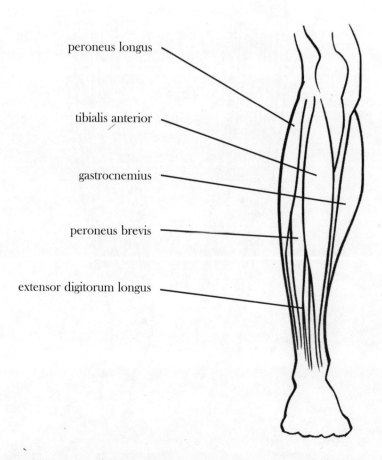

peroneus longus

tibialis anterior

gastrocnemius

peroneus brevis

extensor digitorum longus

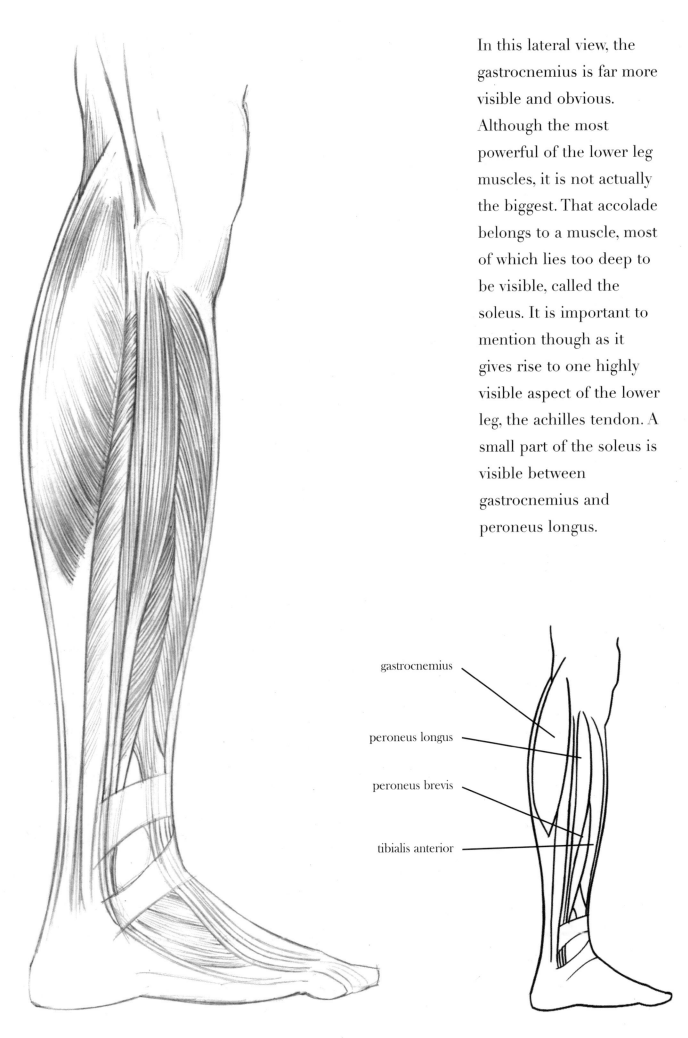

In this lateral view, the gastrocnemius is far more visible and obvious. Although the most powerful of the lower leg muscles, it is not actually the biggest. That accolade belongs to a muscle, most of which lies too deep to be visible, called the soleus. It is important to mention though as it gives rise to one highly visible aspect of the lower leg, the achilles tendon. A small part of the soleus is visible between gastrocnemius and peroneus longus.

gastrocnemius

peroneus longus

peroneus brevis

tibialis anterior

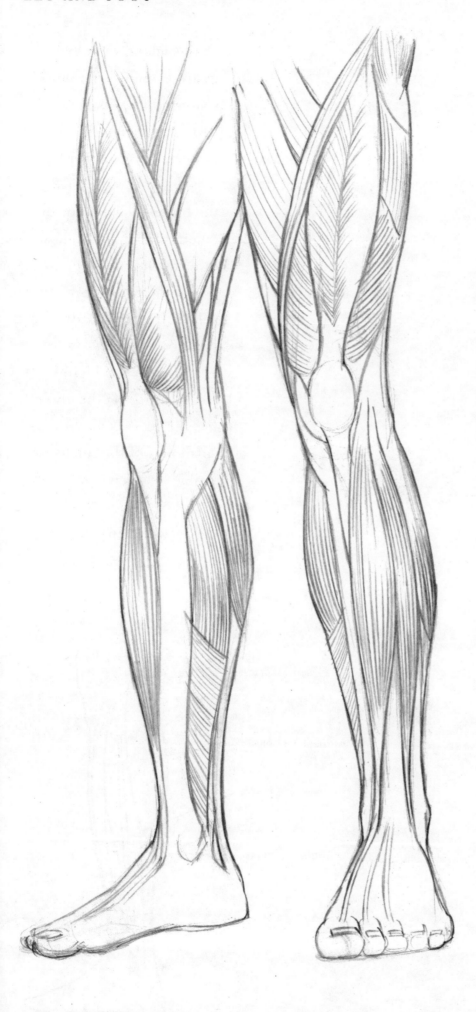

The illustration at left gives us a good overview and should allow us to fill in any gaps as we attempt to complete our mental picture of the legs.

Although missing some tendons and some muscles too deep or too small to warrant inclusion, you should now be able to easily identify all of the major flexors and extensors shown here.

As with the arm, the flexor and extensor muscles which operate the toes lie very deep until they reach the ankle, resulting in a sudden glut of tendons. It's a good idea to prioritize those which are likely to protrude in normal use, e.g. the previously mentioned tibialis anterior.

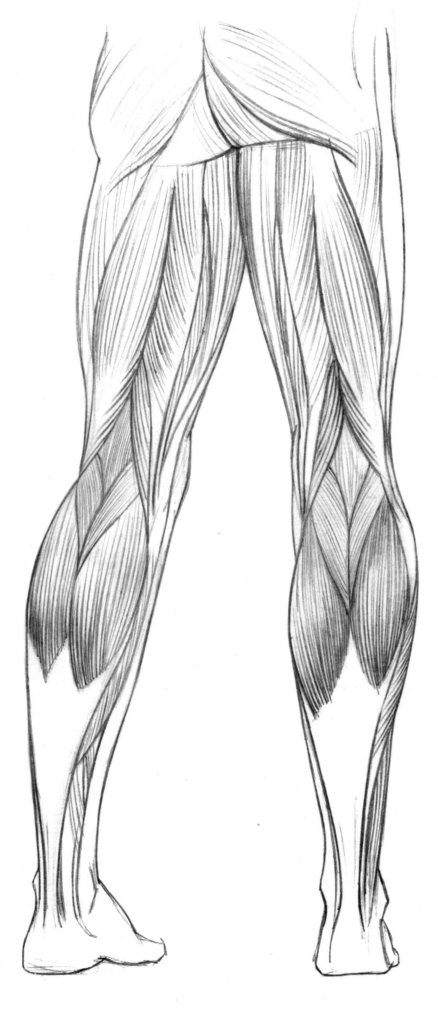

In this rear view of the whole of both legs we can clearly see the highly distinctive pattern produced by the gastrocnemius muscles meeting the biceps muscles of the upper leg. The diamond shape can be an extremely useful tool when working out muscle placement. The hugely powerful flexor muscles of the back of the thigh are divided into two sections: the lateral section being the *long head* and the medial section the *short head*.

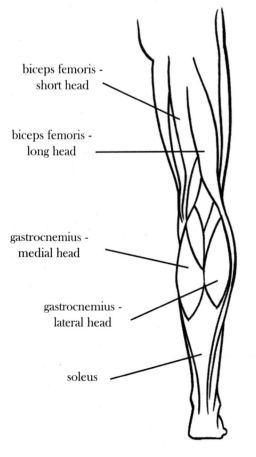

biceps femoris - short head

biceps femoris - long head

gastrocnemius - medial head

gastrocnemius - lateral head

soleus

BONES OF THE FOOT

Although there are obvious similarities between the skeletons of the foot and the hand, we should remember that they have markedly different functions to perform. The heel is first and foremost a load bearer and the foot is situated at approximately ninety degrees to the leg. From a component point of view however, the foot bones are of a similar design to those of the hand. The collection of small bones immediately in front of the heel are the *tarsal bones* and correspond with the carpal bones of the hand.

Likewise the foot has metatarsal bones and phalanges.

The great load bearer, the heel is unsurprisingly the largest bone of the foot and has the latin appelation of *calcaneus*. Situated on top of this sits the *talus*. It is the talus that articulates with the *malleoli* or ankle bones of the lower leg, with a surface that allows a high degree of articulation.

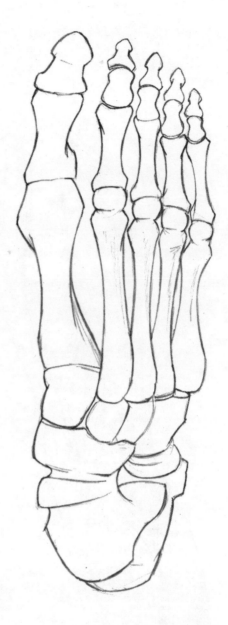

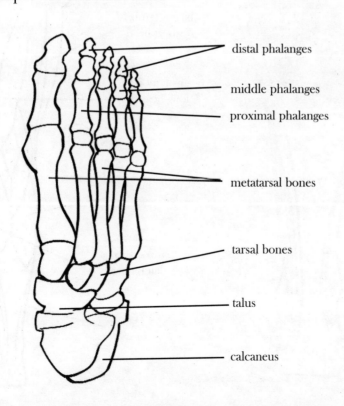

distal phalanges

middle phalanges

proximal phalanges

metatarsal bones

tarsal bones

talus

calcaneus

In this lateral view of the bones of the feet, we can clearly see the mass of the heel, or calcaneus. It's also clear the part it plays in the arch of the foot. The complex, only semi-tight connection to the metatarsals allows the foot to have a fair degree of 'give'. This is essential given it's need to bear large weights, as a slightly flexible series of bones is far less prone to breaking than a single, inflexible one.

Articulating with the tarsal bones are the *metatarsals*, making up much of the length of the foot. These terminate in ball-like heads which in turn articulate with the first row or proximal phanlanges. As with the thumb, the toe has only two phalanges, with the middle phalanx being absent. As a result, the two it does have are far more massive than any of those of the toes.

The phalanges and metatarsals are named first through fifth from the big toe to the little toe respectively.

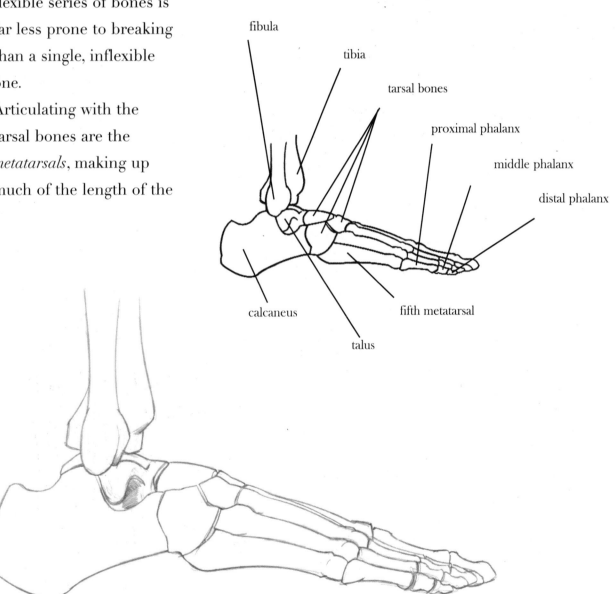

fibula

tibia

tarsal bones

proximal phalanx

middle phalanx

distal phalanx

calcaneus

fifth metatarsal

talus

MUSCLES OF THE FOOT

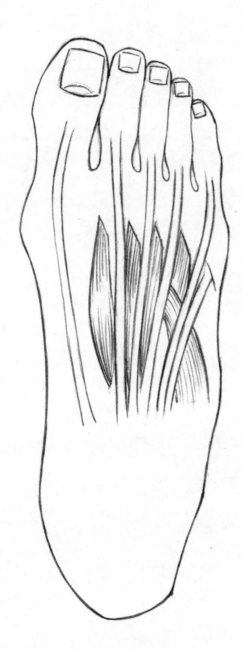

It should be immediately obvious to anyone looking at the top of their own foot that there is precious little in the way of muscle to talk about. The exceptions are the group of small muscles seen at left known as the *dorsal interosseous* muscles, *dorsal* because they are on the top of the foot and *interosseous* because they are situated between the bones. Also visible is part of *extensor digitalis brevis* which originates at the calcaneus and divides into four tendons attaching to the toes deep beneath the surface. Lying just above the bones are the tendons of *extensor digitorum longus*, used in straightening the toes. The tendon running to the big toe is from *extensor hallucis longus*. It's worth noting at this point the direction which the toes tend to point. It may or not be from millenia of wearing footwear, but our toes have a tendency to point inwards, rather than projecting outward in a straight line.

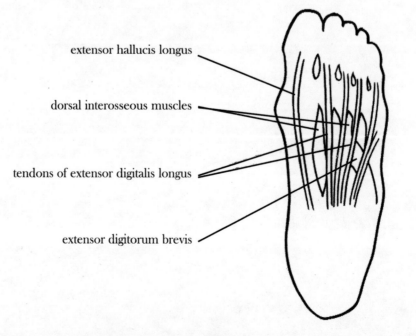

extensor hallucis longus

dorsal interosseous muscles

tendons of extensor digitalis longus

extensor digitorum brevis

In this lateral view of the foot we can more clearly see *extensor digitorum brevis.* Behind and below the malleolus of the fibula run two tendons. These are the tendons of the extensor muscles mentioned on page (102), *peroneus brevis* and *peroneus longus.* They are held in place by the tape-like *peroneal retinacula,* which also restrains other tendons at the ankle. *Peroneus longus* reaches and attaches to the fifth metatarsal.

Also clearly visible is the achilles tendon, or to give it its proper name, *tendo calcaneus.* As detailed earlier, this tendon emanates from the soleus muscle deep within the lower leg, attaching to the heel or calcaneus.

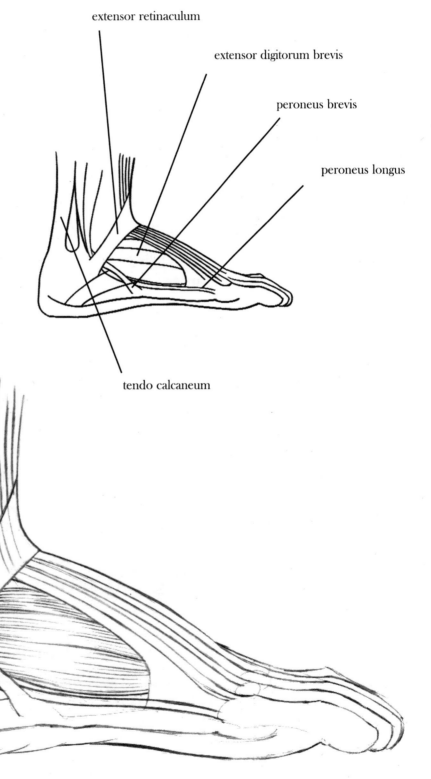

extensor retinaculum

extensor digitorum brevis

peroneus brevis

peroneus longus

tendo calcaneum

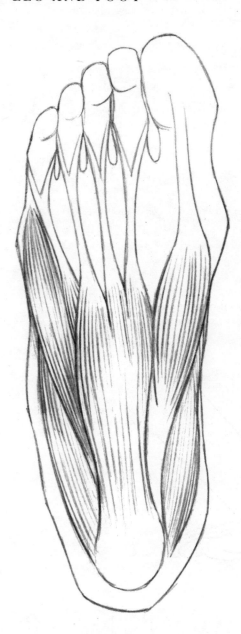

The sole of the foot is where we find the bulk of the muscles. Emanating from the calcaneus and dividing into tendons attaching to the phalanges of the toes this is the *flexor digitorum brevis* muscle, used to curl the toes. To the lateral side of this is the *abductor digiti minimi*. This too originates at the calcaneus and attaches to the base of the little toe. On the medial side lies the *abductor hallucis*, which again has its origin at the calcaneus. It runs the length of the foot and inserts at the base of the big toe.

Above this and to the right of flexor digitorum brevis is *flexor hallucis brevis*. This muscle originates at the tarsal bones and connects to the base of the big toe.

Overleaf: As with the lateral view, on the medial side a tendon runs behind and below the the malleolus. In this case it belongs to *flexor hallucis longus*, originating from the fibula and running all the way to the distal phalanx of the big toe.

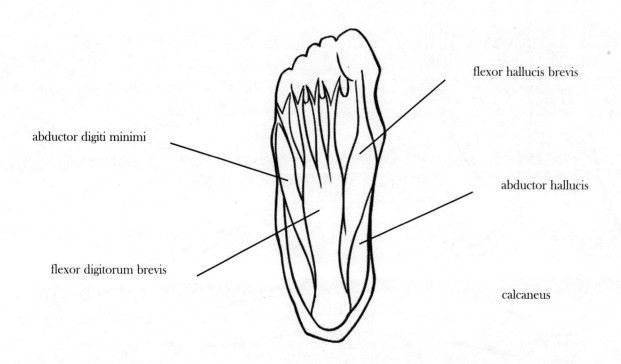

abductor digiti minimi

flexor hallucis brevis

abductor hallucis

flexor digitorum brevis

calcaneus

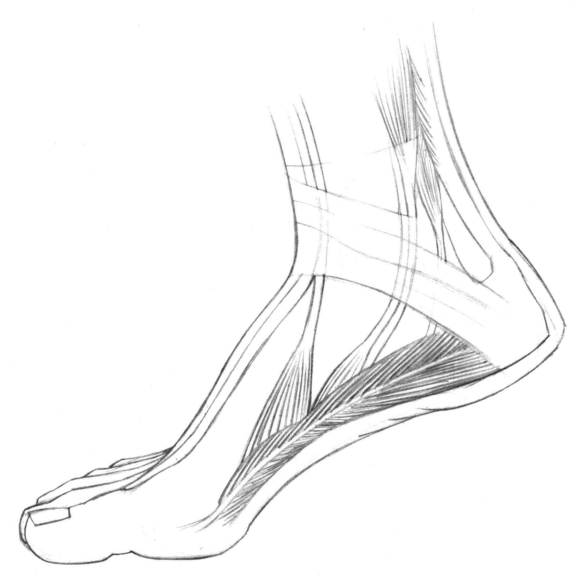

In the illustration above we can also clearly see both the *entensor retinaculum* and the *flexor retinaculum*. These fibrous ribbons are essential for holding the bundles of tendons in place. Although they are not actually visible on the surface, their effects certainly are and as such help to inform our decision making. Understanding all of the mechanics makes us all better artists.

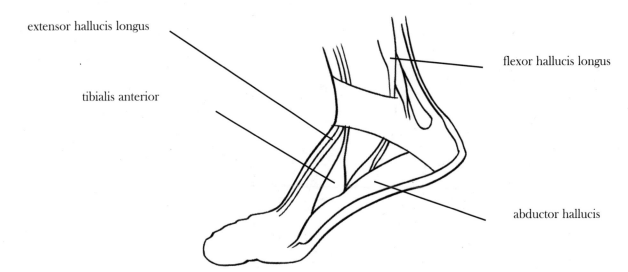

extensor hallucis longus

tibialis anterior

flexor hallucis longus

abductor hallucis

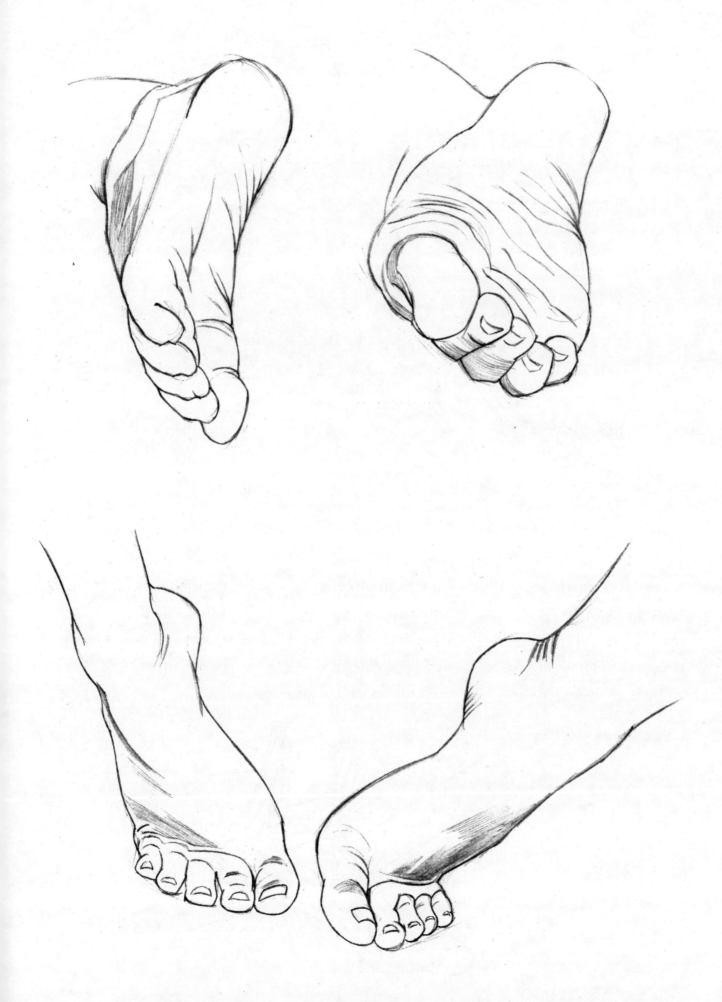

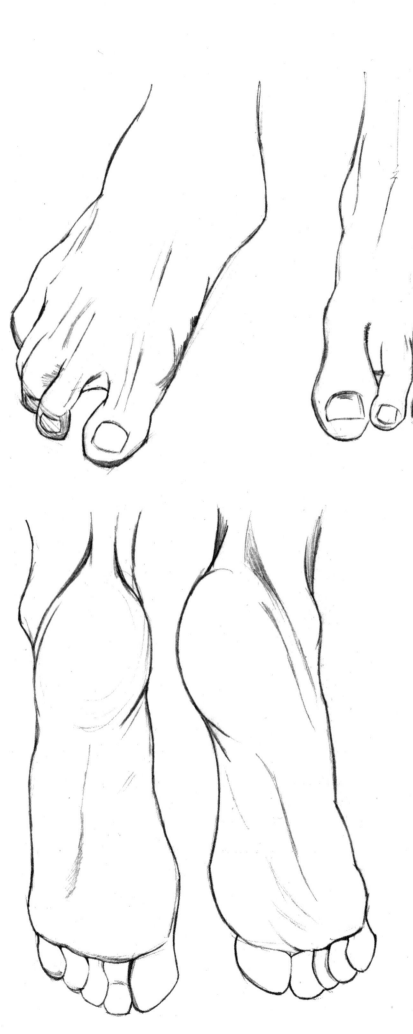

Foot Studies
These studies of feet all give us different information about changes in the surface form given different angles and uses of the foot.

At top left I've drawn the feet head-on, upside-down and at a three-quarter view. Forcing ourselves to try the unusual is the only way to make discoveries.
In the drawing above, the toes take on a gripping quality almost worthy of the hands.

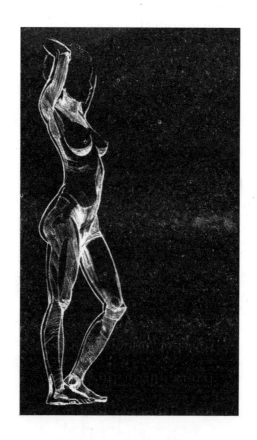

REAL PEOPLE

REAL PEOPLE
Form and surface

Knowing the skeletal framework and the muscle system of the human body is essential. But all of this will do us little good if we ultimately can't put it all together to form convincing figure drawings. That's what this chapter is all about.

Drawing the complete human form requires extra disciplines in subjects such as weight, light, surface texture, foreshortening and many more. Each of these subjects is worthy of a whole book to themselves, but for now we'll concern ourselves with the chief points only.

The figure to our right is both balanced and relaxed; the pelvis and spine have just the right amount of tilt to make us believe the model could maintain this pose for a prolonged period. It should be stating the obvious to say that the vast majority of her weight is on her left leg. This in turn means that her upper body has to have the weight distributed so as not to cause imbalance. Move her shoulders just a little to her right and she will begin to look as though she may topple over. Also, the position of her left leg tells us that it is 'locked', using the natural limits of the flexibility of the knee joint to steady her. This provides a very strong basis on which to support a body.

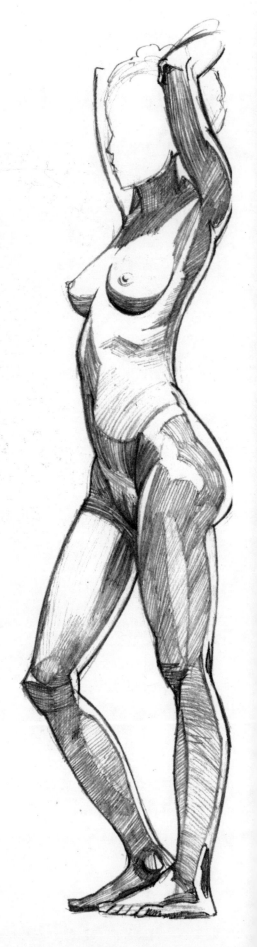

116

Although the figure on this page is in a kneeling position, weight is still important to consider. We have to be convinced that the figure's buttocks are resting out his outturned feet.

There is also a high degree of contrast in the light used in this drawing. This has a large bearing on the viewers perception as to the position of the various parts of the body. It is not simply the outline of the figure which is giving us this information, it is also the light falling on the figure. Form is described by showing which parts of the body are turned towards the light and which parts lie in shadow.

Needless to say, our light source has to appear to be consistent. If the light falling on one part of our model appears to be coming from a different direction to the light on a different part, this will not only confuse the

viewer, it will completely undermine the form of the figure we are studying.

The effect light has when it strikes any surface is worthy of a lifetimes work - ask the impressionists!

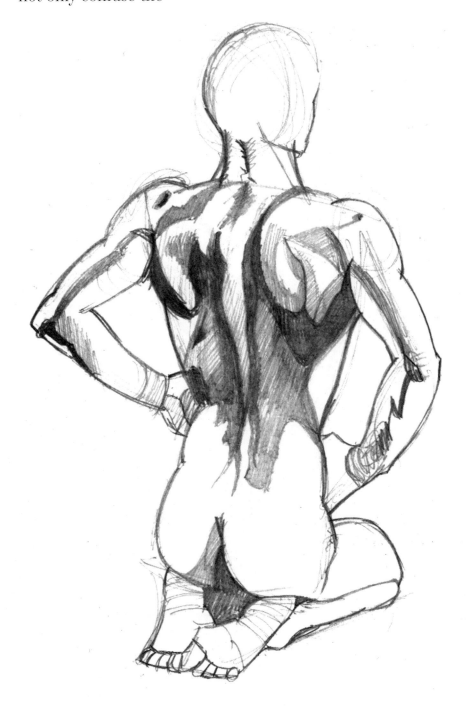

Mapping the Superficial

When we consider the surface of any form we should look for indicators that tell us not only that we believe what we're seeing but also why we believe it. Subtle changes in direction of the most minute details of, say, the creases of the skin can be all it takes to describe the contours of the body. The area of the upper buttock and lower back in the image below uses this idea. The lines on the figure mirror the journey that the models own skin may take. The same technique has been used on the foreshortened leg at the bottom right. Indications of surface shape of this kind all help the viewer in 'reading' the image and creating depth in their own minds.

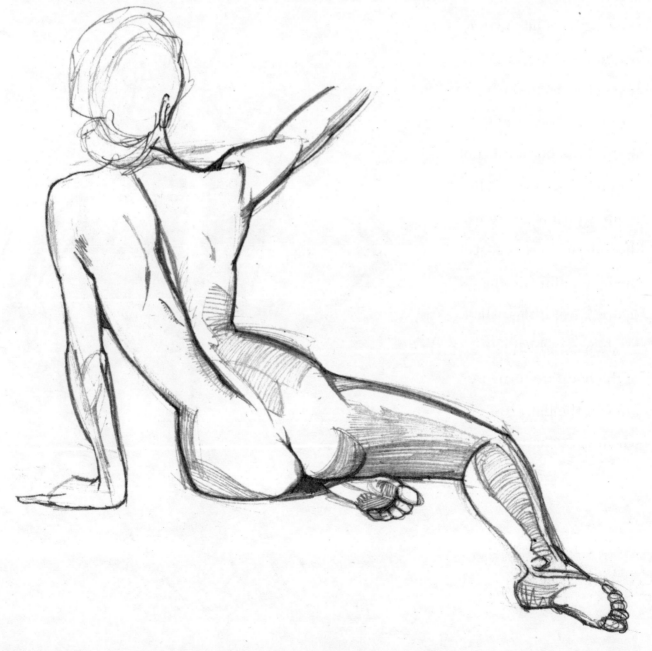

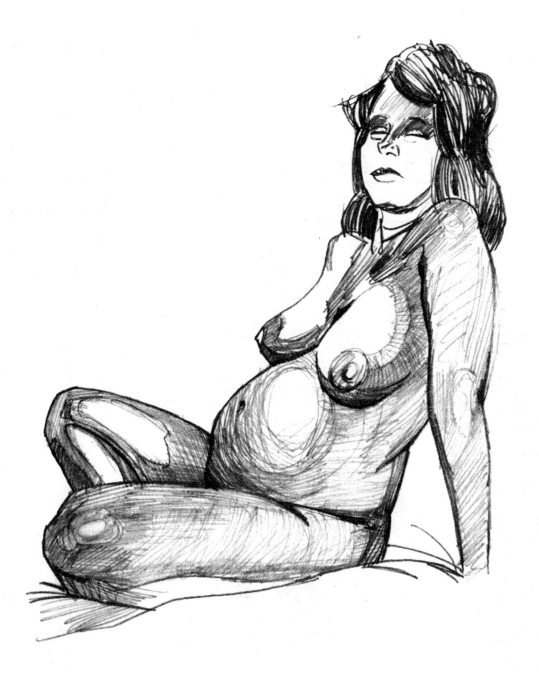

The above drawing takes this technique even further. A pregnant woman is an ideal subject for this kind of study, given the forms which need to be described. This is a study of both light and surface. Any area which is not saturated with light has been described with directional lines. These have been kept deliberately loose, as a tighter approach can soon look very contrived. Remember, this is a study and as such should be used as an information gathering exercise and not necessarily an attempt to create a finished masterpiece.

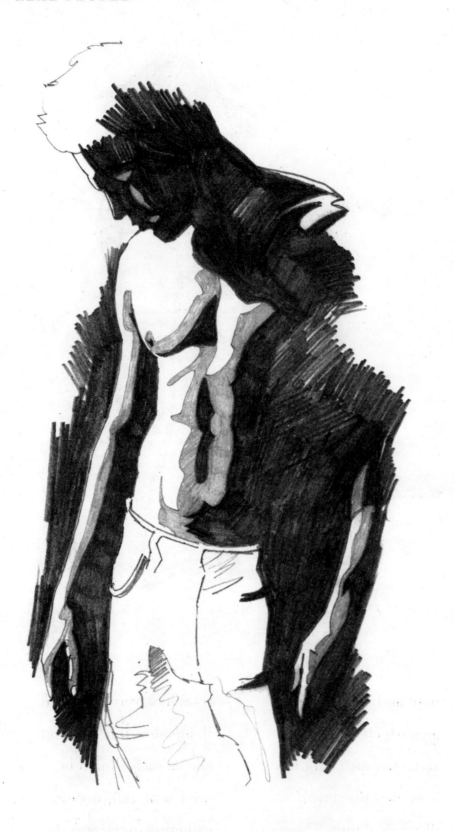

the figure is well observed and backed up with an understanding of anatomy we can recreate complex forms with just a few simple lines. This requires very careful observation and as much of a knowledge of what to leave out as what to include.

If we chose to take this principle much beyond the drawing at right, it would begin to become abstract. This may well produce some interesting results, but would not be particularly instructional for a book on anatomy.

These drawings use a strict discipline, allowing only three tones to describe the form. We can set ourselves any challenge we think may yield results along these lines. The parameters we set will depend ultimately on what it is we are hoping to achieve.

The two drawings on these pages rely on pure light to reveal the human form. There are no outlines, only a variation in tone to indicate three states of light: pure light, neutral light and pure darkness.

It is often surprising how much we can say about the human body with just a minimum of information. If

Light plays a vital role in
figure drawing: multiple
light sources create a much
greater level of subtlety,
producing often unexpected
challenges. Single light
sources however, throw the
figure into stark relief and
for this reason are a good
choice for the learner.
If the light source is very
close to the subject, there
will be a marked difference
in contrast between the
points nearest and furthest
from the light. Try drawing a
figure posed with their head
directly beneath the light.
This will have the effect of
bringing out the prominent
features of the skull.
No one should be surprised
to learn that the drawing on
the right was made from a
single light source, or have
too much difficulty
discerning the direction of
that source.

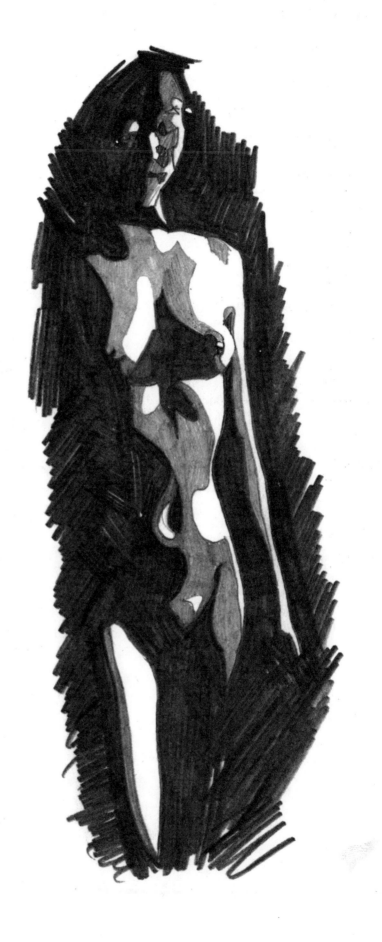

CLOTHING

Given that most people
aren't usually walking
around naked, it's only
right that we should
devote some of the
remaining space to talk
about clothing.
Given the enormous
range of fabrics available
we'll have to confine
ourselves to speaking
generally. There are basic
guidelines for drawing
clothing effectively, so
let's stick to these.
The two extremes of
clothing are on the one
hand fabric so thin and
close-fitting as to take on
the effect of an extra layer
of skin, and on the other,
so heavy and voluminous
and to more or less bury
the physical attributes of
the wearer.

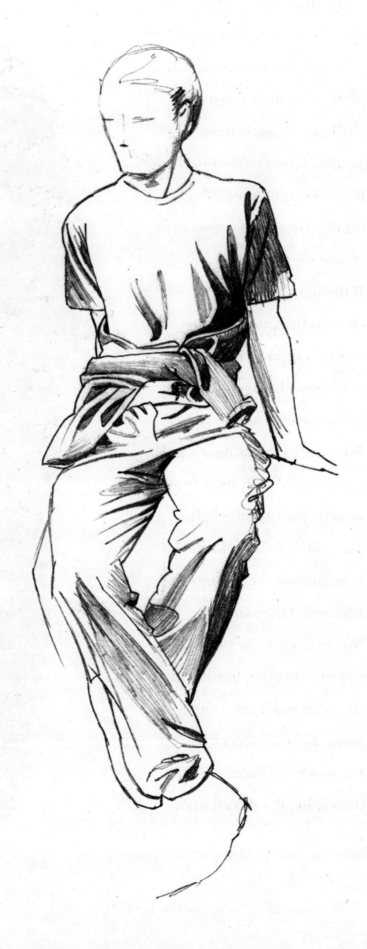

Simple and light

A t-shirt is as good a place as any to begin our look at clothing. T-shirts are very unfussy in their design and their fabrics come in a range of thicknesses.

The one to our right is of a fairly light fabric. This makes the incidence of folds and creases much higher than if the fabric were, say, leather. What causes the folds and creases? Much as the skin of our bellies will tend to form folds as we bend over, so will any fabric. Keep in mind that fabric folds have a points of origin and destination and that these points are usually based at or around the areas of highest stress. In the case of this particular garment, these points are the armpit, the breasts and the belly, but often

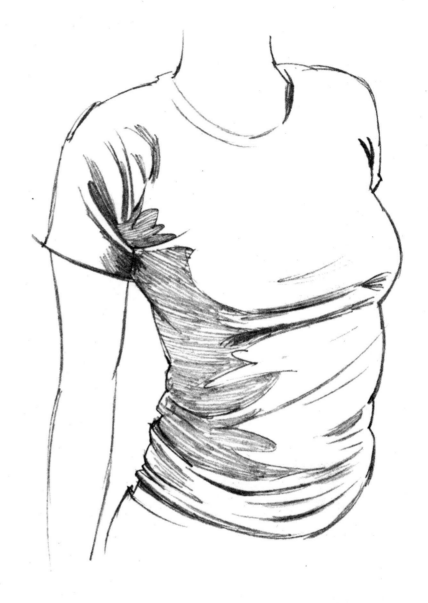

also include the elbow, the shoulders and the neck.On the lower body the crotch, knees and ankles are usually the source of twisting, folding and creasing.

Try to make sure that the lines you produce make sense as a whole and remember their purpose as far as drawing is concerned is to 'point' to the areas mentioned.

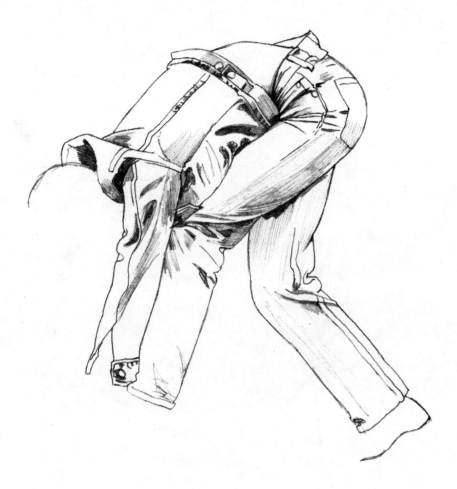

twisting, just an extreme compression of fabric as the weight of the model's torso bears down on its upper ridge.

Look at the detail and notice the fact that the back of the jeans are nowhere near the model's lower back. This is typical of an unyielding, heavy material such as denim. It is this kind of unexpected detail which puts the credibility into our drawing.

Here we have a study of the effects of putting a heavy fabric, in this case denim, under high stress. Particular attention has been paid to the area in front of the pelvis. All of the lines which follow the gluteal area appear to be converging, just out of sight in the pubic area. This is what I meant by 'pointing' on the previous page.

In many ways, this is reminiscent of something we've seen earlier - the point adjacent to the armpit where the pectoral muscle inserts. Here though, there is no

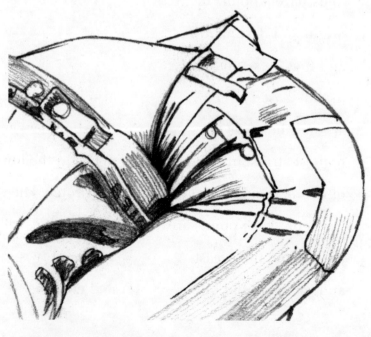

Loose Fit

Let's have a look at the way much looser clothes hang on the body.

At right is a sitting figure wearing a heavy, long-sleeved sweater and loose, heavy fabric jeans. She also has a coat draped over her lap. There is very little in the way of small creases here, as the thick fabric will only allow this if pushed to extremes. Even then, the creases can be no nearer than double the fabric's thickness because a crease is, in essence, the result of the material being doubled over. Below is an even more extreme example. Our model is wearing a heavy robe which does not lend itself to either many or

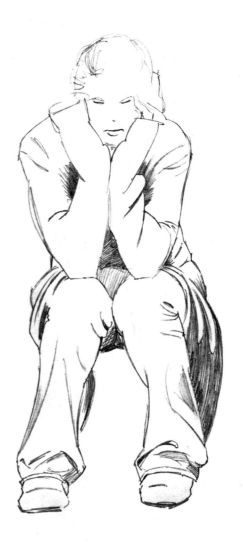

highly pronounced folds. On a fabric this thick, lines tend to be rounded off and lack many, if any harsh or sudden changes in direction.

To really learn the difference, try persuading a friend to sit for you in the same pose twice, wearing first the lightest top available, followed by the heaviest.

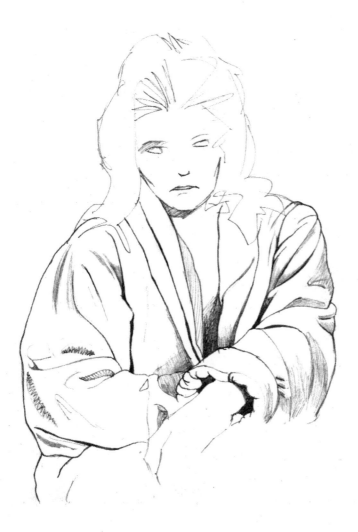

A Glossary of Terms Used in this Book

Anterior	frontal
Aponeurosis -	a fibrous, sheet like membrane particularly for holding tendons in their proper place.
Bicep	a large, twin tendoned flexor muscle of the upper arm.
Clavicle	more commonly known as the collar bone, running between the sternum and the shoulder
Condyle	a rounded, protruding, articular surface of a joint
Cranium	The larger, upper section of the skull
Deltoids	the muscles of the shoulder
Dorsal	top, or viewed from above
Femur	also known as the thighbone, the long, single bone of the upper leg.
Fibula	the smaller of the two bones of the lower leg
Humerus	The single bone of the upper arm
lateral	side, outlying
Ligament	a tough, flat fibre holding bones together.
Mandible	also known as the jawbone, the smaller, lower section of the skull
Mastoid	a prominent neck muscle running between the base of the cranium and the sternum
Medial	side, inlying
Pectoralis	a muscle of the chest
Posterior	rear
Radius	joining laterally at the elbow, one of the two lower arm bones
Scapula	two roughly triangular plates covering the upper back and joining the shoulder
Serratus	a group of small muscles running from the scapula to the ribs

Sternum	also known as the breastbone, the flattish, central bone at the anterior of the ribs
Tendon	the narrow insertion section of a muscle
Tibia	the larger, weight supporting bone of the lower leg
Torso	joining medially at the elbow, one of the two arm bones
Trapezius	a large, quite flat muscle of the upper back and neck
Tricep	a three tendoned extensor muscle of the upper arm
Trochlea	a spool-shaped protrusion on the elbow joint of the humerus
Tuberosity	a bumpy, raised or rough area on a bone which allows tendons to gain purchase
Ulna	joining medially at the elbow, one of the two lower arm bones
Vertebra	one of the bones comprising the spine. pl. *vertabrae*